Clean Eating Made Simple

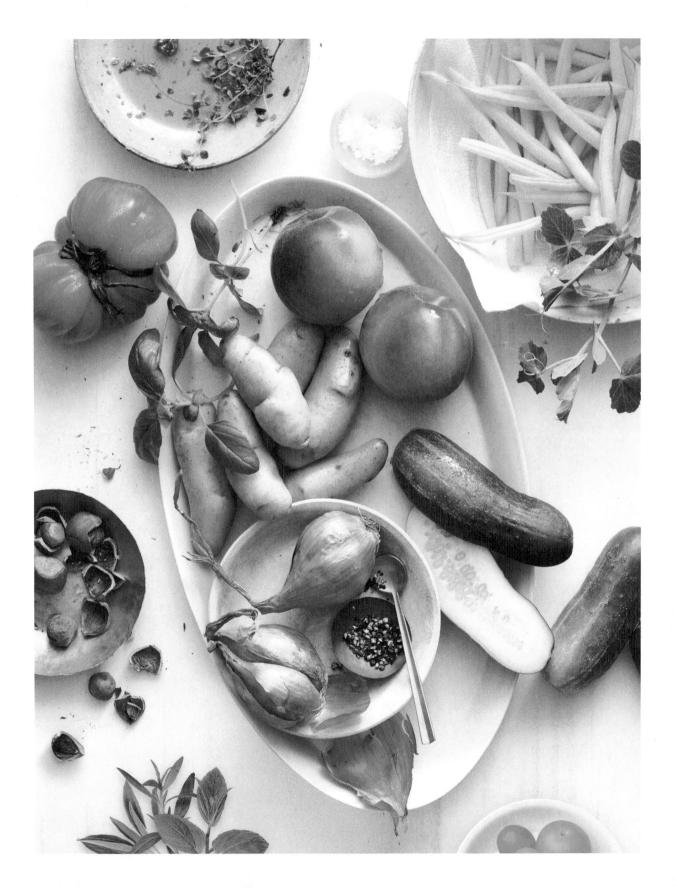

Clean Eating
Made Simple

A HEALTHY COOKBOOK WITH DELICIOUS WHOLE-FOOD RECIPES FOR EATING CLEAN

**ROCKRIDGE
PRESS**

Contents

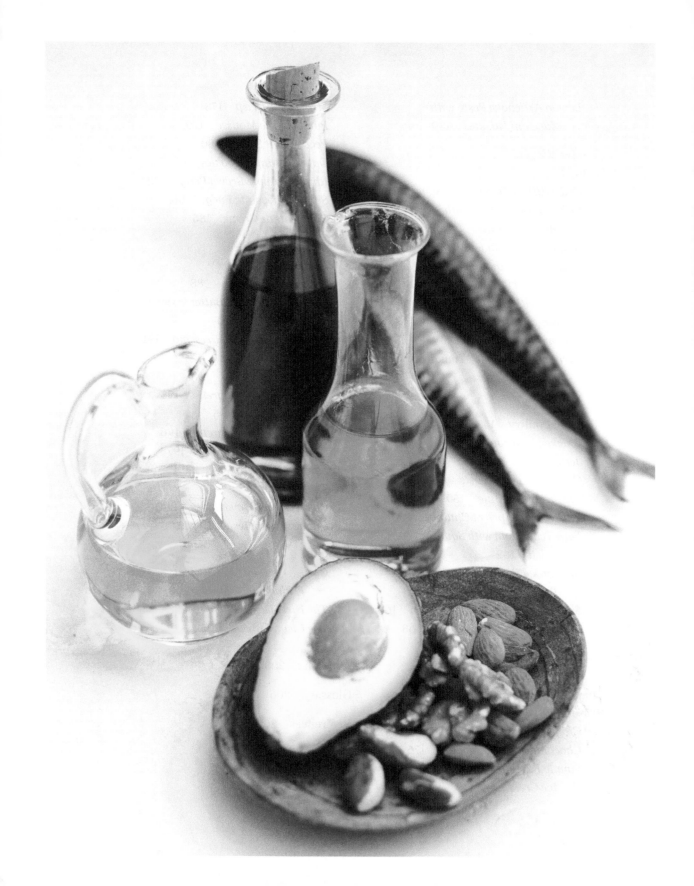

Introduction

What did you eat for breakfast this morning? More importantly, how much of that meal contained actual nutrients? It seems like a simple question, but eating has become a complicated subject. Although the majority of consumers are more informed than ever before, more information has not necessarily created healthier eaters.

Several decades ago science began to bombard people with recommendations about what nutrients to eat for long-term wellness. The problem with this proliferation of research is that recommendations kept changing, leaving people more confused than ever about what to eat. Every day another study pinpoints a specific benefit of a nutrient—we're talking about you, *acai* berries—and people scramble to add doses of these nutrients into their diet, at least until the next transformative study comes along.

Riding closely on those scientific proclamations are the food manufacturers peddling processed foods to concerned consumers in the name of good health. The push to alter foods that were already nutritious has led to the average North American consuming approximately 150 pounds of food additives a year. This slide towards processed products started decades ago, and a dwindling of real food in supermarkets made it difficult to make healthy choices. If you glance at the aisles in the grocery store the labels lead you to believe that nearly every item is a healthy choice—think organic, gluten-free, low-fat, sugar-free, added vitamins, fibers, and nutrients, the list goes on. The truth is, if you eat whole foods you get a dose of nutrients in their most beneficial state, their natural state, no added nutrients needed. The idea that water requires extra doses of vitamins and nutrients is laughable; it already *is* a nutrient.

Fortunately, a back-to-basics clean eating food movement is on the menu du jour. Clean eating is simple; it eliminates additives by promoting natural, whole foods with an emphasis on fresh, seasonal produce. The rules? Eat foods in their natural state. Eat food that looks like food—it's not that complicated.

Clean eating involves taking a closer look at the quality of the products you consume. Is what you ate for breakfast a meal that nourishes and sustains your body? Everything needed to support a strong immune system, prevent chronic disease, and provide the energy required to live a full active life can be found in the clean eating diet. The added bonus of this lifestyle choice is that the ingredients are delicious, easy to find, and will actually accomplish what food is supposed to do, nourish you.

Clean Eating Made Simple provides the basic principles to clean eating without overcomplicating your diet. A guide back to the basics, you'll learn the fundamentals of the clean eating diet, discover tips and techniques to easily implement the clean eating plan into your daily lifestyle routine, and start enjoying delicious recipes.

Eating doesn't have to be so difficult. Best conveyed in the words of Michael Pollan, food activist and author of *In Defense of Food, The Omnivore's Dilemma*, and *Food Rules*, "Don't eat anything your great-grandmother wouldn't recognize as food."

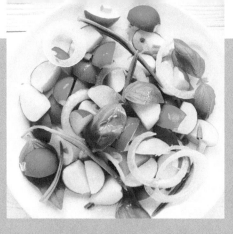

Clean Eating Basics

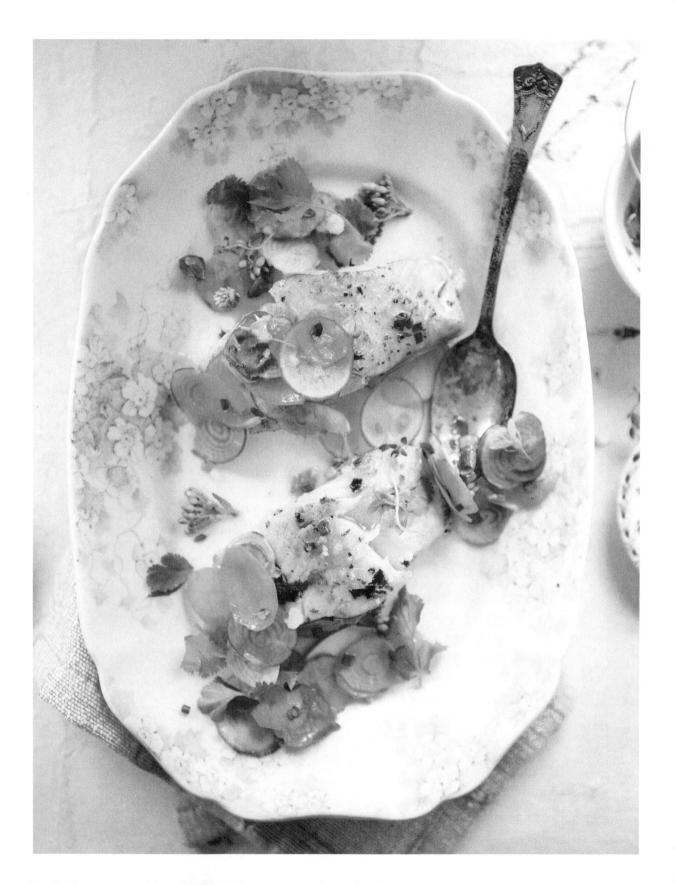

CHAPTER ONE

Fundamentals of Clean Eating

Clean eating does not have a specific definition because it is not a specific diet. Clean eating is choosing to live your life in a healthier way. Choosing to eat clean means filling your plate with natural, wholesome foods and excluding anything processed or refined. The idea is not deprivation in the interest of weight loss, as with some other diets, but rather rediscovering and embracing fresh, unaltered food that nourishes your body.

Your relationship with food will forever change when you understand that what goes on your plate is fuel for your body. The quality of fuel directly affects the way your body performs, so why not provide the best possible food choices through clean eating?

Your clean eating plan will follow certain principles, such as eating smaller, more frequent meals and staying hydrated, but the plan is flexible and you are an individual. A clean eating plan will not be the same for everyone. Life happens, and if you can eat clean at least 80 percent of the time you will reap wonderful health benefits and feel energized.

What Is Clean Eating?

Clean eating was not a mainstream diet and lifestyle plan before Canadian fitness model Tosca Reno introduced her version of clean eating in a series of books. This plan gained almost instant acceptance, especially among those trying to lose weight, because Tosca herself went from fat and frumpy to sleek and toned following clean eating principles.

Clean eating did not originate with Tosca Reno though. The concept as a whole was first popular in the 1960s counterculture as another form of rebellion against corporate encroachment in almost every facet of life. People rejected the proliferation of processed food that was part of a conformist, middle-class lifestyle, and they embraced natural, whole foods instead. This clean eating movement was furthered by several books exposing the dangers of pesticides and food additives and the effects they had on human beings and on the food chain.

During this clean food activism period, another group of people quietly and successfully used the same principles, without the political element, to get healthy and fit. To them, clean food equaled more energy and quicker muscle recovery and growth, as well as overall good health. This group consisted of bodybuilders and weightlifters. It is this subculture that Tosca tapped into when joining the weightlifting scene under the advice of fitness publisher Robert Kennedy, whom she eventually married.

Although she didn't invent clean eating, Tosca has pared the concepts down to simple guidelines that produce results, and that people can follow easily. Clean eating should never be considered a fad diet or even a temporary diet. It is meant to be a lifestyle that includes food and exercise to succeed.

Clean Eating Principles

So now that you know how clean eating came about, it is time to look at what guidelines you will follow on the plan. Remember, your goal can be 100 percent clean eating, but following these simple principles even 80 percent of the time will enable you to reap all the health benefits of the plan. This is a long-term lifestyle choice. Try to be practical and flexible with your food and exercise goals. It gets easier as time passes and you develop new habits.

Eat Whole Foods, Such as Whole Grains, Lean Proteins, and Fresh Fruits and Vegetables

Whole and fresh foods are at the foundation of the clean eating diet. Eat a variety of delicious fresh foods that are as close to their natural state as possible. "Whole" does not mean an entire orange or head of lettuce; it means unrefined and unprocessed. Processed foods are stripped of valuable nutrients, pumped full of additives, and can contribute to disease and poor health. There are some packaged items that can still be clean foods, but a good basic rule is that if you don't recognize an ingredient or can't pronounce it, you probably don't want to eat it!

Eat Five to Six Small Meals a Day

Many people grew up with the notion of three square meals a day with no consideration given to individual body requirements or the ill effects of spiking and plummeting blood sugar. A good, steady influx of nutritious foods can regulate and stabilize blood sugar, creating fewer food cravings for sugar or caffeine and supplying you with energy throughout the day.

Eat Every Two to Three Hours and Never Skip a Meal

The principle of eating meals regularly and frequently goes hand in hand with eating smaller, more frequent meals to avoid blood sugar fluctuations. You might think that skipping breakfast or starving yourself through lunch is a good way to lose weight or control your diet. Unfortunately, all you are doing is creating a massive blood-sugar tsunami that will eventually crash, wreaking havoc on your body. Start your day with a wholesome breakfast to kick-start your metabolism, and top up the tank every few hours afterward.

Drink at Least Eight Cups of Water a Day

Keeping your body hydrated is a healthy diet staple for most eating plans, and is good common sense. Your body is about two-thirds water and needs water for everything to work correctly and efficiently. Water helps flush toxins from the cells and tissues, helps in the absorption of nutrients, and regulates body temperature. Always have a bottle of water on hand and sip from it throughout your day. If you are thirsty, your body is already dehydrated.

Eat Healthy Portion Sizes

In a supersized world it is important to realize that you might be eating more than you need, which can contribute to weight gain and poor health. When you first start eating clean, you may not know what the right portion size is for a chicken breast or bowl of cereal. Weigh and measure your food until you can eyeball it accurately. If you don't have a scale, most clean eating portions can be measured roughly using your hands. Fruit and vegetable portions should just about fit into your two cupped hands (1½ cups), starchy carbohydrates should fit in one cupped hand (¾ cup), and lean protein portions should be about the size of your palm (6 ounces).

Combine Lean Protein and Complex Carbohydrates in Every Meal

Pairing protein and carbohydrates is a cornerstone of the clean eating diet, because this combination of food groups is extremely effective for stabilizing blood sugar. The slow release of sugar into the blood, rather than the quick rush created by carbohydrates or protein alone, can also help burn fat and promote healthy weight loss. So try a couple of apple slices with a small scoop of natural nut butter or wrap a lean piece of chicken in a whole-grain tortilla for lunch, and see how much better you feel.

Avoid Refined, Processed Foods

The list of foods to avoid might seem long, but once you start eating clean, those refined and processed foods will no longer be the least bit appealing to you. The list includes candy, white bread, white rice, lunch meats, pizza, cookies, processed cheese, junk food, and even products that are labeled as healthy, such as low-calorie frozen dinners.

Eliminate Sugar

You should avoid refined sugar like the plague because that is exactly what this poison can be, deadly. Refined sugar can cause devastating effects such as diabetes, high blood pressure, obesity, depression and fatigue. While your body uses glucose converted from foods as energy for every process in the body, the type of sugar that is found in processed foods is fructose. When you consume fructose the entire burden of processing it falls on your liver, creating waste products and toxins. There is more to purging sugar from your diet than not buying sweet cereals. The best defense to avoid refined sugar is to read food labels carefully, even on clean foods such as Greek yogurt. If you see words ending in "ose" or "sweetener" beware, this is usually sugar in disguise. If you need a little sweetness in your meals, add naturally sweet fruits and vegetables.

Include Healthy Fats and Eliminate Unhealthy Fats

Fat has become the enemy in many healthy eating circles, but this should not be the case, because your body needs healthy fats to function. Healthy fats (monounsaturated fats and polyunsaturated fatty acids) help synthesize hormones, provide fuel for the body, and assist in the absorption of some vitamins. Many clean eating foods contain healthy fat such as avocado, salmon, olive oil, and eggs. The unhealthy fats (saturated fats and trans fats) contribute to obesity, heart disease, diabetes, and other health issues.

Never Leave Home Without Clean Eating Foods

One of the main reasons people fall off the healthy-eating wagon is they find themselves stranded in a sea of processed products and fast food when they are away from home. When you are hungry and your blood sugar is plummeting, it is hard not to give in to the plethora of unhealthy choices surrounding you. The solution is a cooler bag filled with clean eating meals and snacks that you can tote with you to work or school. This portable clean eating "cornucopia" will also ensure you don't skip meals. You can even pack all your foods the night before, for convenience.

The Benefits of Clean Eating

Many people have a combative relationship with their food, due to years of fluctuating weight and poor health, as well as eating products that are processed and simply bad for you. It can be difficult to understand that food is supposed to make you feel energized. There should be no side effects from a great meal. Clean eating will forever change how you perceive food because the benefits of this lifestyle will be evident in your mirror and in your body after a very short time on the plan. Depending on your initial physical state and commitment to clean eating, you might experience some of the following benefits sooner than others.

General Feeling of Well-Being

Eating nutritious, healthy food and avoiding foods clogged with fat, sugar, and preservatives will make your body feel great. How could it not, when all the building blocks of good health are sitting on your plate? There will be a spring in your step, and you will feel motivated to continue on your clean eating journey.

Better Immune System

An effective disease-fighting immune system starts with the food you eat, especially colorful fruits and vegetables packed with vitamin C, other antioxidants like beta-carotene, plus vitamins and minerals. Vitamin C can increase the number of antibodies and white blood cells available to fight off disease and infections. Zinc can also increase white blood cell counts.

Improved Sleep

Sleep is a crucial component of good health, and lack of sleep can have serious detrimental effects on the body. All the nutrients found in clean eating foods help stabilize and regulate the hormones responsible for supporting deep sleep at night. There is also a definitive link between sleep deprivation and obesity. Getting seven to eight hours of quality sleep a night can also help with your weight loss goals.

Increased Energy Levels

Many people rely on the artificial, fleeting energy rush they get from either caffeine or sugar to get through the day. This artificial high is usually followed by a crash that requires another unhealthy boost, which creates a vicious cycle and a tired body. Clean eating provides a sustained slow energy boost that comes from a steady release of sugar—achieved by combining proteins with complex carbohydrates and fiber, as is found in Greek yogurt and fruit. This combination provides energy all day with no midmorning or midafternoon crash.

Healthy Hair and Clear Skin

The first areas of the body that suffer when you are not getting enough nutrients in your diet or are eating too much harmful food are often you hair and skin. They are like a barometer of good health. Whole, clean food and adequate hydration will flush harmful toxins and free radicals from your body, creating a youthful glow and lustrous, healthy hair.

Improved Mental Clarity

Your brain is like any other organ in the body: It needs a steady influx of vitamins, fats, proteins, essential fatty acids, and minerals to help it run well. Clear thought, mental alertness, and decreased fatigue are all results of clean eating. The high level of antioxidants in produce may also help protect the brain from the ravages of Alzheimer's disease and dementia.

Decreased Body Fat

Many people start the clean eating diet to lose weight, and while clean eating is not a weight-loss diet, losing weight is a natural result of eliminating empty-calorie processed foods and eating whole, nutritious foods. All the foods you avoid when eating clean are key contributors to obesity. All the foods you eat—clean, healthy food—will fill you up and stop food cravings without adding empty calories to your body.

Decreased Risk of Cancer, Heart Disease, and Diabetes

Cancer, heart disease, and diabetes are the major causes of death around the world. These diseases can be prevented by diminishing their common risk factors, which include obesity, high blood pressure, high blood sugar, high cholesterol, and a sedentary lifestyle. All these risk factors are decreased when eating clean.

Improved Mood

Depression and mood disorders can have their roots in vitamin and nutrient deficiencies. Increased availability of vitamins and minerals through healthy eating can improve mood. Some whole foods also contain vitamins that help produce mood-elevating chemicals in the body, such as dopamine from vitamin B_6 contained in sunflower seeds and cooked tuna. Also, when you are energized and maintain a healthy weight, you will feel attractive and confident.

Prevention of Age-Related Ailments and Conditions

Many debilitating diseases associated with old age are preventable with healthy clean eating. No matter when you start eating clean (in your twenties, fifties, or even seventies), your body will respond by becoming the efficient machine it is meant to be. Providing the right fuel can keep joints lubricated and pain free, improve mobility, and help create a positive outlook well into the golden years.

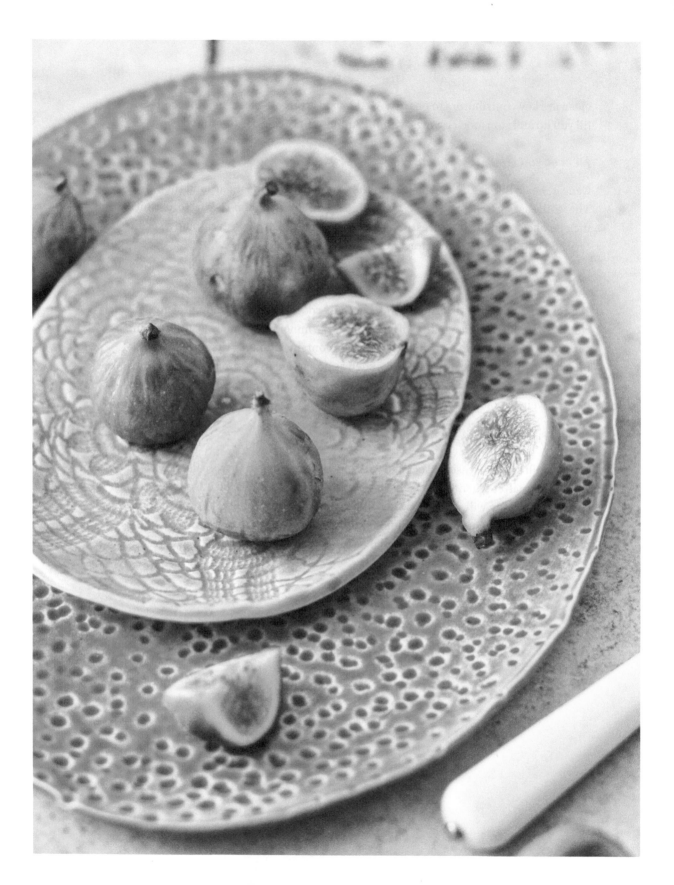

CHAPTER TWO

Clean Eating Foods

Many diets are all about what you can't eat in the interest of losing weight, but clean eating is about the abundance you *can* eat with vibrant good health as a goal and weight loss as a nice bonus. The foods included in this lifestyle are as close to their natural form as possible, with no additives, refining, or processing. You will be eating from every food group, even healthy fats, and not counting each calorie you put in your mouth.

Every food has a unique and valuable complement of nutrients that serve important functions in the body. This means variety is the key when meal planning and shopping. You will be reading labels and sourcing the best products possible from butchers, fishmongers, and farmers' markets. This might sound like a big commitment, but you will soon be making clean eating choices easily as they become a habit. The goal is to gravitate toward craving fresh blueberries rather than blueberry muffins and a handful of tasty almonds rather than salty potato chips. The supplements and nutrients your body needs already exist in food in their most natural form.

Don't worry if you do have an occasional clean eating lapse, such as eating a slice of your mother's famous pecan pie. Clean eating is a long-term lifestyle, which means perfection is not practical. Simply enjoy the moment and then go back to the numerous natural food choices that nurture your body.

What's On the Clean Eating Diet?

You will be delighted to see how many delicious foods are on the clean eating list. This is not a comprehensive list, but a guideline to give you an idea of the choices available. The bulk of your diet should be fruits, vegetables, whole grains, lean proteins, and healthy fats.

Foods to Include in Your Diet

- All fruits, fresh and frozen
- All vegetables, fresh and frozen
- Almond milk
- Applesauce, unsweetened
- Baking powder
- Baking soda
- Brown rice cakes
- Canned tomatoes (sodium-free)
- Canned tuna and salmon (packed in water)
- Chicken breast (skinless, boneless)
- Cocoa powder
- Coffee
- Cooking spray, fat-free
- Cream cheese
- Dried fruit
- Edamame
- Eggs, organic free-range, if possible
- Feta cheese, low-sodium
- Fish (except the ones considered to be high in mercury)
- Game meats (elk, venison, bison, buffalo, rabbit)
- Granola (homemade or unsweetened store-bought)
- Grass-fed beef, trimmed
- Greek yogurt, plain
- Green tea
- Ground beef, extra lean
- Ground chicken, lean
- Ground lamb, lean
- Ground pork, lean
- Ground turkey, extra lean
- Herbal teas
- Herbs and spices
- Hot sauce
- Hummus
- Lamb rack
- Legumes (black beans, black eyed peas, chickpeas, lentils, kidney beans)
- Kefir
- Ketchup (organic, low-sugar)
- Mustard
- Nuts (in smaller amounts)
- Nut butters (in moderation)
- Nut flours
- Nut milks
- Nutritional yeast

- Olives
- Pickles
- Pork chops or roast, trimmed
- Pork tenderloin
- Protein powder (all-natural)
- Pure vanilla extract
- Salsa
- Sauerkraut
- Seafood (lobster, crab, scallops, clams, mussels, shrimp)
- Sea salt
- Seeds (chia, sunflower, flax, pumpkin, sesame)
- Skim milk
- Soba noodles
- Stock, low-sodium, fat-free (vegetable, beef, chicken)
- Tahini
- Tofu and tempeh
- Turkey breast (skinless, boneless)
- Veal
- Vinegars (apple cider, rice, balsamic)
- Whole grains
- Whole-grain breads, pitas, tortillas
- Whole-grain flours (whole-wheat, oat, quinoa, amaranth, spelt)
- Whole-grain pasta
- Whole-wheat bread crumbs
- Yogurt, plain

Foods to Cut Down on or Use Sparingly

These are foods that are still considered to be clean, but due to their fat, sodium, or sugar content (naturally occurring), they should be used in small amounts in the cooking process or as an ingredient.

- Avocado oil
- Coconut oil
- Fruit juices
- Grapeseed oil
- Honey
- Maple syrup
- Olive oil
- Pumpkin seed oil
- Sea salt
- Stevia
- Sunflower oil
- Tamari or low-sodium soy sauce
- Unsalted butter
- Walnut oil

Foods to Eliminate

This list contains refined or processed items that you need to stay away from to reap the benefits of clean eating. Eliminate any food that contains these items as ingredients. Also eliminate any food that has ingredients you don't recognize.

- Alcohol
- Artificial sweeteners
- Chocolate spreads
- Foods high in saturated fats or trans fats
- Frozen dinners
- Fruit drinks and cocktails (not labeled as juice or 100 percent juice)
- Hydrogenated oils
- Junk foods
- Marshmallow spreads
- Processed meats
- Preservatives
- Soda
- Sugar
- White flour
- White pasta

What's the Problem with Processed Foods?

People eat much more processed food than they realize. Many would be horrified if they added it all up for a typical day. Processed foods are convenient, designed to taste good, and difficult to avoid. One of the problems with processed foods is the lack of information about what happens to the food before it hits the grocery shelf—and worse, what it does to your body. Since processed foods have become the bulk of most people's diets, the prevalence of diseases such as obesity, heart disease, diabetes, and cancer have skyrocketed.

Food processing sounds like it should be relatively simple: Take raw ingredients and turn them into food products that are safe to eat. Unfortunately, processed foods are changed to the point where they are almost unrecognizable—all in the interest of a longer shelf life, approved food safety, and supposed enhancement of the natural product. Some processed foods still make the clean eating list, particularly if you "process" them yourself. Freezing and dehydrating are great preservation methods that do not change the nutritional makeup of the original food very much. Look for frozen foods that are flash frozen with no additives and for dehydrated foods that have no preservatives or sugar added.

Unfortunately, most commercial processing techniques affect the raw natural ingredients catastrophically. Processing strips food of nutrients, phytonutrients, flavor, moisture, and texture. Some processing techniques are designed to add these lost components back into the food, along with preservatives, dyes, synthetic flavors, stabilizers, anti-caking agents, emulsifiers, humectants, fats, and sugars. When you consider these extra ingredients, processed food suddenly does not look as appetizing. These many changes to the food turn it into something unnatural to the body, and that can create major health issues.

Some of the reasons to avoid eating processed foods include:

- **Chronic illness and general poor health.** Many diseases are caused by chronic inflammation in the body. Inflammation is a natural response of the body to something that is damaging. Unfortunately, this inflammation cycle can become destructive to the body itself when the damaging agent is constantly reintroduced or the immune system starts to attack healthy tissue. Heart disease, cancer, asthma, Crohn's disease, arteriosclerosis, dementia, neurological problems, and rheumatoid arthritis have all been linked to chronic inflammation. Many studies (a host of them published in the *American Journal of Clinical Nutrition*) have shown that refined flour and sugar, vegetable oils, and other additives in processed foods cause chronic inflammation.

- **Addiction to processed foods.** This is a huge bonus for food manufacturers, because you start craving processed foods and purchase more. This addiction is caused by the fact that ingredients in processed foods increase your body's production of a pleasure neurotransmitter called dopamine.

- **Genetically modified ingredients.** Many processed foods are made up of genetically modified ingredients. They are not usually included on clean eating plans because they are not considered to be completely natural. How delicious does your corn cereal taste when you know it was initially created in a laboratory?

- **Weight gain.** Common ingredients in processed foods, such as high-fructose corn syrup and hydrogenated vegetable oil, are conclusively linked with obesity.

- **Negative effects on mental health.** Spiking blood sugar from sugary processed foods and nutritionally substandard ingredients can create mental fog, mood swings, an inability to concentrate, fatigue, depression, and headaches.

- **Increased aging.** Phosphate additives in processed foods can contribute to loss of bone density, kidney disease, and accelerated aging of the cells in the body.

Clean Eating Food Groups

Clean eating is not about eliminating any one food group. You will see carbohydrates, proteins, and fats in the meal plans and recipes in this book. In most cases you will not have to go out of your way to get enough fat in your diet, because healthy oils such as olive oil, as well as the oils that occur naturally in products like peanut butter, are used in recipes in recommended quantities. There is a great deal of flexibility in the clean eating food groups, so you will never feel deprived or hungry.

Complex Carbohydrates

How many servings should you eat?

Six to ten servings a day (55 percent of your diet; made up of 35 percent dietary fiber and 20 percent starchy carbs)

What are complex carbohydrates?

The carbohydrates you eat are found in two forms: simple and complex. Complex carbohydrates are the type that is consumed on the clean eating plan, except for a few simple carbs in the form of some fruit. Complex carbohydrates consist of at least three sugars held together to form a chain. These chains don't create a quick rise in blood sugar because they take longer to digest. There are two types of complex carbohydrates: starches and dietary fiber. They are found mainly in fruits, vegetables, nuts, seeds, and grains.

What do they do in the body?

Complex carbohydrates are used for fuel in the body. When you eat carbohydrates, either simple or complex, the body breaks them down into sugar to use as fuel. When the sugar levels in the blood rise, the pancreas produces insulin, which stimulates the cells to absorb the sugar, causing blood sugar levels to fall again. If blood sugar levels fall too low, the pancreas produces a hormone called glucagon that prompts the liver to release stored sugar into the blood. This delicate balancing act ensures that the cells of the body have a constant supply of energy. The glycemic index is a tool used to rank carbohydrates based on how much and how fast the blood sugar levels rise after eating a food. This scale ranks food from 0 to 100, with foods scoring between 0 and 55 considered to be low on the glycemic index. This is the range where most complex carbohydrates fall.

Benefits

Complex carbohydrates are required primarily in the body as fuel, powering all the body's functions. If you don't eat enough of them, you will experience fatigue, mental fogginess, mood swings, and irritability.

They also have other benefits. The fiber in these foods improves digestion. Fiber is the part of the complex carbohydrate that is not digested. It acts as a broom sweeping through your digestive system. This fiber pushes the food through the system, along with other undigested substances and toxins. Complex carbs also contain important vitamins, minerals, phytonutrients, and antioxidants. These nutrients are crucial to help prevent most diseases and keep the body as healthy as possible.

Dangers

Some people experience problems when eating certain complex carbohydrates if they are sensitive to gluten, a protein found in cereal grains. This sensitivity manifests as celiac disease or gluten intolerance. Gluten causes an atypical immune response that can cause damage in the lining of the small intestine, creating unpleasant symptoms and malabsorption of nutrients.

Shopping guide

When you are eating clean, most of your shopping cart should be filled with complex carbohydrates, because this group includes fresh produce, nuts, whole grains, and multigrain pastas and breads. Try to buy your fruit and vegetables locally and in season, paying particular attention to their freshness and ripeness. Also consider buying organic whenever possible, especially for the items on the Dirty Dozen list created every year by the Environmental Working Group, which ranks the amount of pesticide contamination in commercially grown produce. Produce on this list contains the most pesticide residue. (Since the list does change a bit from year to year, it's worth checking it out yourself at www.ewg.org/foodnews/summary.php. They also put out a Clean Fifteen list (page 205) that shows the least contaminated produce.) Local co-ops, farmers' markets, and even your own garden are the best places to find great clean eating fruits and vegetables.

Whole grains can be purchased year round and can be found in the bulk section of most supermarkets. When you get your grains home, you will need to store them more carefully because they have healthy oils in them. Store your whole grains in airtight containers in a cool, dry place or in the freezer for up to six months.

Lean Proteins

How many servings should you eat?

Five to six servings a day (27 percent of your diet)

What are lean proteins?

Protein molecules are made up of amino acids held together by peptide bonds. Proteins perform a wide variety of functions within the body and are also the building blocks of cells. Twenty amino acids are required to synthesize protein, and each type of protein is made of an exact combination of amino acids in a certain order. Nine of these amino acids cannot be synthesized in the body, so they must come from the food we eat. Amino acids cannot be stored, which means you need to consume them in your diet to meet the daily needs of the body.

What do lean proteins do in the body?

A better question might be, what doesn't protein do in the body? Protein plays a part in almost every function in the body. Some of the roles protein plays include:

- Carrying oxygen in the blood
- Making antibodies
- Helping muscle contract and move
- Making enzymes
- Making hormones
- Acting as neurotransmitters
- Storing iron in the liver
- Building, repairing, and strengthening cells, protective coverings, and connective tissue

Benefits

Since protein is essential to so many functions in the body, it is obvious that eating it has many benefits. Beyond supporting all the bodily functions and general good health, including lean protein in your diet can help build muscle after a hard workout by repairing and rebuilding the muscle. Eating protein supports weight loss by helping you feel full longer. Eating lean protein instead of proteins that are loaded with saturated fats can cut the risk of heart disease by lowering cholesterol and blood pressure levels. And protein helps boost the immune system.

Dangers

There are problems with both too little and too much protein, as well as eating proteins that contain too much fat. Too little or poor-quality protein in your diet can create a deficiency that may cause poor digestion, water retention, repressed immunity, slow wound healing, hair loss, and, in severe cases, liver damage. Diets that are too high in protein can increase the risk of osteoporosis and cancer, put a strain on the kidneys, and create a nutritional deficiency. The reason *lean* proteins are the clean eating choice is because the saturated fat in fattier protein sources can contribute to cancer, heart disease, diabetes, and other health problems.

Shopping guide

Clean eating proteins include a broad range of foods. The most common protein sources are meats, poultry, fish, seafood, and eggs. Protein can also be found in dairy foods, grains, nuts, seeds, and vegetables, although most vegetables need to be combined with other types of food to create a complete protein that contains all nine essential amino acids.

When shopping for meats, get the freshest, leanest cuts possible. Look for meat with little fat marbling and trim off any excess fat before using it in your recipes. Go for skinless chicken, or take the skin off yourself and trim any visible fat. When buying fish or seafood, do your homework on what types are caught locally or in season and make sure it is fresh. Your fish should never have a strong scent or be slimy.

Grains, nuts, and seeds are an important part of the clean eating diet, so try to buy your staples in bulk whenever possible to save money. Store these products in sealed containers in the refrigerator or freezer to keep them fresh longer.

Healthy Fats

How many servings should you eat?

Two to three servings a day (18 percent of your diet)

What are healthy fats?

Fat is an essential nutrient that provides energy, helps the body function, and helps other nutrients do their jobs. There are four kinds of fat—two associated with eating clean and two to be avoided. The two healthy fats allowed in moderation on the clean eating plan are monounsaturated fats and polyunsaturated fats, which include omega-3 and omega-6 fatty acids. The two unhealthy fats to be avoided are saturated fats and trans fats.

What do healthy fats do in the body?

The healthy fats allowed on the clean eating diet have many functions in the body. These include:

- Providing a source of immediate and stored energy
- Helping the body absorb fat-soluble vitamins, such as vitamins A, D, E, and K
- Insulating the body
- Providing essential nutrients cell function and repair
- Helping regulate blood sugar
- Promoting mental clarity and memory retention
- Playing a crucial part in hormone production

Benefits

Healthy fats have a great many benefits in the body. Despite the bad reputation fat has in general with the healthy eating community, healthy fat can:

- Decrease your risk of heart disease and type 2 diabetes
- Help prevent belly fat
- Protect against irregular heartbeat
- Improve good cholesterol levels
- Improve blood pressure
- Help prevent plaque build-up in the arteries
- Strengthen the immune system
- Support healthy skin

Dangers

Many people don't realize that the danger associated with fat is specific to the type of fat and amount consumed. You will be eliminating saturated fat and trans fat from your diet, so health issues associated with those fats will be minimal. Healthy fats still represent a danger if you eat too much of them. Consuming more monounsaturated fat than is recommended can lead to weight gain, although it will not increase your risk of heart disease. Too much polyunsaturated fat can lower good (HDL) cholesterol and increase your cancer risk.

Shopping guide

Healthy fats are found in many types of foods, including vegetable oils, nuts, seeds, some fruit (such as avocado), and fish. Buying fresh is the key to great fish. Research the varieties that are local or in season in your area, or find a knowledgeable fishmonger who can point you in the right direction. Fish with high mercury levels, such as fresh tuna, shark, swordfish, and orange roughy, should be eaten infrequently to limit your exposure to the metal. (To learn more about which fish have the highest and lowest mercury levels, check out the Natural Resources Defense Council's guide at www.nrdc.org/health/effects/mercury/guide.asp.)

Take a careful look at the bottles of oil on your grocery shelf. Make sure the seals are tight and there isn't any dust on them. The oils should also be stored out of direct sunlight and away from heat sources. Nuts and seeds can be purchased in bulk and stored for several months in sealed containers either in a cool, dry place or the refrigerator.

As for oils, clean eating oils include:

- Almond oil
- Avocado oil
- Coconut oil
- Extra virgin olive oil
- Unrefined safflower oil
- Unrefined sunflower oil
- Unrefined walnut oil

Clean eating oils *do not* include:

- Canola oil
- Corn oil
- Hydrogenated oil
- Palm or palm kernel oil
- Vegetable oil

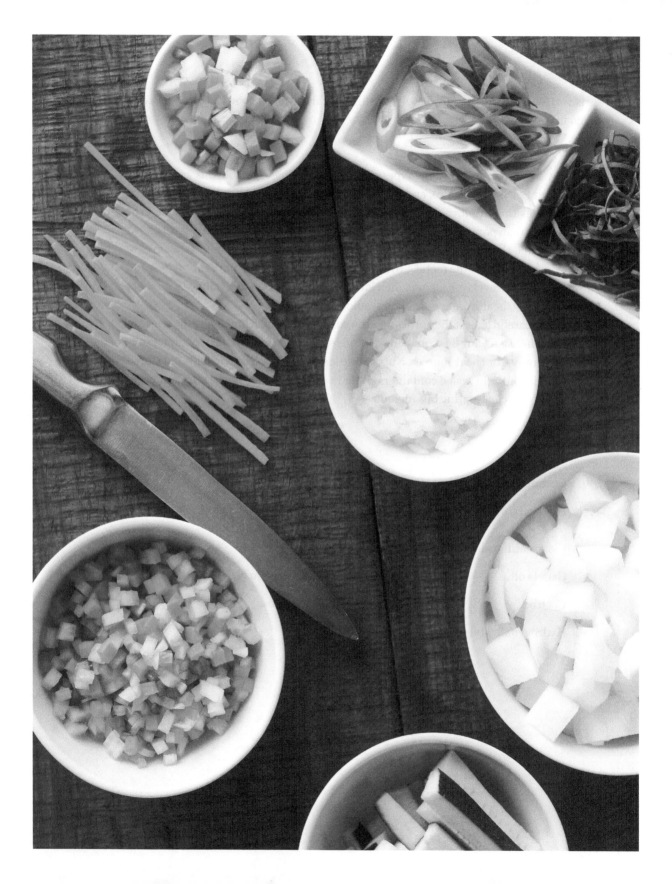

CHAPTER THREE

Everyday Clean Eating Plan

You will have well over a thousand opportunities a year to choose clean eating and support your healthy lifestyle. If you eat five small meals a day, every day that's 1,825 meals each year! That's a lot of meals to organize, so it is clear that meal plans are crucial for success. Fortunately, with so many delicious natural ingredients to choose from in the pantry and the refrigerator, clean eating meal plans are flexible. This means your meal plans can take your lifestyle and diet into consideration.

Meals consisting of nutritious, unprocessed food are only part of a successful clean eating strategy. You also have to consider exercise. A healthy body requires regular exercise to function effectively, and clean eating includes exercise, both cardio and weight training, as an integral component. Plan for a minimum of thirty minutes of exercise a day, four days a week, in your daily clean eating routine.

Make a Weekly Plan

An important part of eating clean is having a meal plan in place each and every week. This is key to ensure that you have clean eating choices on hand at home and when you go to work or school. The plan's flexibility allows for leftovers or eating out on occasion, as long as you follow the general parameters as outlined in chapter one. A typical clean eating day, whether omnivore or vegetarian, should include the following:

- Five to six small meals, spaced out every few hours (no skipping meals) to guarantee stable blood sugar levels; these meals are breakfast, lunch, and dinner, with two or three snacks in between

- Appropriate portion sizes

- A minimum of eight glasses of water, with water as the main drink in your plan

- A combination of complex carbohydrates and protein in each meal, including snacks

- Healthy fats, because fat is not the enemy as long as it makes up no more than 18 percent of your calories

- A focus on eating fresh, natural, high-quality food; everything else will fall into place

People have different palates, health conditions, and schedules. This means the typical clean eating meal plan will be slightly different for each person, even when following the basic guidelines listed here. Remember, there is no set food per meal, beyond combining complex carbs and protein.

A Day in the Life of a Clean Eater

Wake Up

Always start your day with a mug of hot water and freshly squeezed lemon juice to detoxify the liver and hydrate the body. This morning routine will be the same for the omnivore and vegetarian meal plans.

Breakfast

Many people skip breakfast in the interest of losing weight or because they are in too much of a hurry to eat anything in the morning. Breakfast is crucial to a healthy body. After sleeping all night, you need to replenish your fuel stores. Also, people who skip breakfast usually crave high-sugar foods later in the day, creating a destructive cycle of blood sugar spikes and deficits. There is no excuse for missing this important meal, especially when you have a clean eating plan in place.

Ten Clean Eating Breakfast Ideas

1. Oatmeal with fresh fruit, chopped nuts, dried fruit, applesauce, or Greek yogurt

2. Breakfast sandwiches with vegetables, eggs, lean meats, or nut spreads

3. Omelets, frittatas, poached eggs, hardboiled eggs (either vegetarian or made with lean meats, fish, or seafood)

4. Low-fat whole-grain quick breads or muffins (made with added protein powder or another protein source, such as almond milk or nut flour)

5. Whole-grain toast with nut butter and fresh fruit

6. Whole-wheat pancakes, waffles, or crêpes (made with added protein powder or another protein source, such as almond milk or nut flour)

7. Greek yogurt with grains, granola, or fresh fruit

8. Smoothies

9. Homemade protein cookies or bars

10. Fresh vegetables with hummus or peanut butter dip

Breakfast Tips

- Eat leftovers from the night before

- Whip up a breakfast casserole the night before and bake it in the morning

- Put oats or grains in your slow cooker overnight for a nutritious, quick breakfast

- Make a tray of frittatas and freeze individual portions; simply thaw and make a handy breakfast wrap

- Layer pretty Greek yogurt fruit parfaits for a special meal

- Make pancakes or clean eating waffles and freeze them for future meals; pop them into the toaster and serve with fresh fruit or Greek yogurt

Lunch

Lunch is often as rushed as breakfast, because people are at work or school, and time is limited. This is why taking a packed clean eating cooler is essential to make sure your food choices are healthy and natural. You should have a nutritious snack about two hours before lunch, so that you're not super hungry or craving sugar. Lunch should recharge you as well as help boost flagging energy and concentration to take you through the afternoon. As with every other clean eating meal, lunch should be a balance of complex carbohydrates, lean protein, and healthy fats.

Ten Clean Eating Lunch Ideas

1. Whole-grain wraps or sandwiches stuffed with lean meat, eggs, vegetables, fruit, whole grains, or nut butters

2. Clean eating soup or stew (combining protein and complex carbs)

3. Vegetable or whole-grain salads topped with lean meats, nuts or seeds, avocado or fruit

4. Whole-grain pastas with a variety of toppings and combinations

5. Leftovers from dinner the night before

6. Cut-up vegetables or fruit with nut butters, Greek yogurt, or hummus

7. Your favorite grilled or broiled protein (chicken breast or salmon) with steamed vegetables

8. Clean eating casserole or baked egg dish

9. A smoothie with some substance, such as added protein powder, Greek yogurt, oatmeal, or avocado

10. Homemade protein cookies or bars with fresh fruit

Lunch Tips

- Bring your favorite salad and stuff it into a pita or wrap

- Make sure your dressings and juicy sandwich toppings are packed separately, or the bread will be soggy

- Cook chicken breasts in bulk and store them in individual bags or containers until you need them for a meal

- Try adding cooked whole grains to your favorite soups and stews instead of noodles

Dinner

Dinner is a meal that should be light but satisfying. Many people consider dinner the biggest meal of the day because the entire family is at the table and it is a time to socialize. But dinner should be no larger than any other main clean eating meal. You can still have a substantial meal, but try to have smaller portions of protein and limited fat.

Ten Clean Eating Dinner Ideas

1. Salad topped with fruit and grains, lean meats, fish, or low-fat dairy products

2. Clean eating casserole or stew

3. Soup topped with Greek yogurt, served with a crusty multigrain roll

4. Whole-grain pasta with tomato sauce or pesto, fresh vegetables, and lean meat, fish, or seafood

5. Stir-fry with tofu or lean meat and vegetables, served over brown rice or cooked whole grains

6. Grilled, broiled, or baked meat, poultry, or fish with whole grains and salad or steamed vegetables

7. Sandwich or wrap stuffed with fish, lean meat, tofu, or low-fat dairy, with whole grains and vegetables

8. Egg dishes

9. Curries and stews

10. Protein- and carb-packed smoothie with a fresh green salad

Dinner Tips

- Make double batches of all your soups, stews, and casseroles and freeze the extra for quick and easy meals the following week

- Invest in a slow cooker and set up your dinner in the morning so it cooks all day

- Have breakfast for dinner

- Try to include vegetarian meals regularly, even if you are an omnivore

Snacks

The importance of snacking is underestimated. If you have ever experienced a mid-morning or midafternoon energy crash, you will appreciate how much your body needs stable blood sugar. Clean eating snacks provide wholesome fuel to keep the body on an even keel. These snacks should be eaten about two hours after breakfast and two hours after lunch. You can also include a snack a few hours after dinner, especially if you tend to eat early, are doing something active, or are staying up later. Snacks should still include lean protein and complex carbs. Carry them in a cooler when you leave home, so you always have them on hand. And you don't have to wait until *exactly* two hours after breakfast or lunch to snack. Listen to your body and have a snack when you are hungry, or your energy and concentration start to lag.

Ten Clean Eating Snack Ideas

1. Cut-up fresh fruit or vegetables with a protein-packed dip (such as hummus or tzatziki)

2. A handful of nuts and dried fruit or trail mix

3. A hardboiled egg and fresh sliced tomatoes or radishes

4. Roasted chickpeas

5. Homemade fruit leathers (see the recipe in chapter six)

6. Whole-wheat pinwheels with vegetables and lean meat

7. Cut-up apple with nut butter

8. Greek yogurt topped with fruit

9. Whole-wheat pita "pizzas" with hummus and cut-up fruit or vegetable toppings

10. Clean eating chia pudding with Greek yogurt and fruit

Snack Tips

- Pack your dips at the beginning of the week in handy two-ounce or four-ounce sealed containers

- Cut up an assortment of fresh vegetables to keep in containers in your refrigerator for quick grab-and-go snacks

- Pop ripe grapes in the freezer in a resealable plastic bag to preserve them as a chilly snack

- Save a bit of lunch or breakfast for a quick snack later in the day

Choose Protein and Carbohydrate Combos

When you're planning meals, the recipes in part two of this book are a great place to start. If you are still not sure about what to eat, try using the table below to pair proteins with complex carbohydrates in your own clean eating meals. Many of the standard clean eating meal plan ideas are also vegetarian options. Consider your specific diet needs when looking at the ideas and tips in this book. This list is not comprehensive, but it should give you a good idea of what you can mix and match.

Complex Carbohydrates
Clean eating granola
Fresh fruit
Fresh vegetables
Hot or cold whole-grain cereals
Legumes
Oatmeal
Seeds
Sweet potatoes, yams
Whole-grain bread, wraps, and pita
Whole grains and grasses (brown rice, buckwheat, bulgur, chickpeas, lentils, quinoa)

Proteins
Cheeses and dairy
Chickpeas, lentils, quinoa, split peas
Edamame
Eggs or egg whites
Fish and seafood
Greek yogurt
Lean meats (beef, pork, game meats, veal)
Legumes
Nuts
Nut milks
Natural nut butters
Poultry (skinless and trimmed)
Seeds
Some vegetables and fruits, such as avocadoes, peas, corn, broccoli, dark leafy greens, artichokes, asparagus, Brussels sprouts, and beets
Tofu and tempeh

Don't Forget About Exercise

Eating clean, wholesome foods is just the start of your healthy living plan. The other component is exercise. Start exercising at least three times a week for thirty minutes per session, and build up to five or six times a week for forty-five to sixty minutes a day. This might sound like a big commitment if you're not exercising now, but your energy levels will be considerably higher when you're fueling your body with clean food, and exercise will be a pleasure. You will not reach optimum health without doing at least the minimum amount of exercise recommended by the plan.

Some benefits of regular exercise include:

- Increased energy
- Improved immune system
- Reduced body fat
- Increased muscle mass
- Better sleep
- Improved libido
- Reduced risk of diseases such as diabetes and heart disease
- Faster metabolism
- Fewer food cravings

It is also important to combine cardio and strength training as part of a balanced exercise approach. The benefits of weight training are incredible, and you will actually be able to sculpt your body, depending on the areas you concentrate on in your workout. Pay particular attention to your core—your abdominal, lower-back, and mid-back muscles—because a strong core will support the rest of your body.

The nice part about building more muscle is that muscle burns more calories, even when you're at rest. Your body will also burn calories faster and more efficiently, facilitating weight loss and maintenance. The cardio component of your exercise routine can be anything that gets your heart rate up and your body moving. You can jog, swim, bike, walk, play with your dog, play a sport, or even dance.

As with any life choice, it is essential to keep the exercise component of clean eating in perspective and at a healthy level. Don't get caught up and overtrain, or you will set yourself back physically and actually jeopardize your health. Remember to rest between your workouts, or at least rest certain body parts so they can recover and get stronger. For example, if you do a back workout on Monday, do not work the same muscle group on Tuesday—work on your legs or chest instead. Balance is the key to getting the most benefits from your exercise regime. It is also important to consult with your health provider before starting any exercise routine.

Clean Eating Tips to Kick-Start Your Diet

1. **Clean out your refrigerator, freezer, and cupboards.** This process might not be too drastic if your eating habits were relatively healthy to begin with, but if you are a junk food addict prepare yourself for a very empty kitchen. Removing all the temptations from your personal space will give you the best chance of starting off right and not falling off the wagon a couple of days later when you stumble upon the old Halloween candy in the back of a drawer.

2. **Make a weekly clean eating meal plan.** Clean eating is about making a mindful, informed choice about the food you are putting into your body. Starting each week with a balanced, prepared meal plan is the best tool for success. You will know what you are eating each day and cooking for each meal. This will eliminate those drive-through fast food meals you grab when you have no idea what you're having for dinner. Meal plans will also make shopping a breeze and cut down on midweek stops at the store.

3. **Make a shopping plan.** Never shop without a plan, because stores are designed to entice you to make impulse purchases. Why do you think sugary cereals are at kids' eye level, and snack foods are found next to the cash registers? A shopping list, with sections for each food group (produce, meat, dairy, and pantry items) will get you through the store quickly and efficiently with no surplus purchases. Never plan to shop right after a workout or a long day at work when you will be hungry and everything will look yummy.

4. **Plan for leftovers.** One of the most efficient cooking strategies to save money and time is to make double batches of all your favorite recipes and freeze the extra portions in sealed containers or plastic bags. Some recipes obviously don't transfer well from the pot to the freezer, but you certainly can double up on most soups, stews, casseroles, and chilies, as well as cooked grains and beans. This will ensure you have clean eating meals available even when you are in a schedule crunch. Simply take a container out of the freezer in the morning and thaw it in the refrigerator all day.

5. **Invest in a food processor.** You can certainly prepare lovely clean eating meals with just a few pots, a knife, and a cutting board, but why not make your life easier? Your processor does not need to be an outrageously expensive model with grinding attachments and twelve speeds. You can find effective midrange machines for a reasonable price and cut your kitchen prep time in half.

6. **Learn to read labels and then pay attention to them.** You might as well accept the fact that your grocery shopping trips are going to be a little longer, because if you pick up a can or package, you will be reading the label. Some clean eating foods will be prepackaged because there are some great items on the market made with clean eating in mind. The majority of your cart will be single-ingredient items such as chicken breasts, vegetables, and whole grains, but you also might want to pick up some dried gluten-free pasta or prepared beans. When reading the label, pay the most attention to the ingredient list—unless you are on a strict diet that limits ingredients such as sodium. Then by all means scan the sodium content first to see if the product passes. On the ingredient list, look to make sure that every item is recognizable and on your clean eating list. If not, put it back and keep looking until you find what you need.

7. **Buy locally grown, in-season produce whenever possible.** Organic produce is also a wonderful idea if you can afford it and live in an area that supports that buying choice. If 100 percent organic is not possible, try to at least buy organic for the foods found on the "dirty dozen" list of pesticide-contaminated produce, to reduce your exposure to toxins. Pick up produce that is in season and grown locally to ensure freshness and optimum nutrition. Produce that sits in trucks on the long haul to various supermarkets loses nutrients in transit. Fresh-picked fruit and vegetables also taste better, which means you will want to eat them! Whenever possible, get your produce at local farmers' markets to save money and be informed about where your food is grown.

8. **Throw out preconceived notions about your meals.** When following the clean eating diet, you will often find yourself eating something for one meal that you usually would reserve for another. There is nothing wrong with having a lovely mixed bean and vegetable salad for breakfast or a plate of oatmeal pancakes for dinner. Food is meant to nourish and delight. Use the entire day as your culinary palette and enjoy unique healthy food creations when you want them.

9. **Learn about clean eating ingredients.** You might already know a great deal about many of the foods found on the clean eating shopping list, such as apples, carrots, or chicken. However, there are also going to be new choices and clean eating substitutions for familiar products that might require a bit of research. For example, cooking clean foods might require using an oil that's different from the one you are used to using. Obviously, you will only be using a little oil, but healthy fats are desirable. It is best to be acquainted with the clean eating choices before shopping, so you know what to look for in the aisles.

10. **Cook your meals from scratch.** If you are one of those people who would rather watch a cooking show on television than wield the knife yourself, plan to spend more time in the kitchen. You might never become an avid cook, but making each clean eating meal from scratch allows you to control and choose the ingredients that end up on your plate. You also might think you don't have time to putter around in the kitchen every day. This is where precise planning will be invaluable. Spend one of your days off cooking the food for the week. Prepare cooked chicken breasts and hardboiled eggs, cut up vegetables that hold well, and freeze portions of your favorite meals for later in the week.

11. **Don't drink your calories.** You might not even realize how many calories you consume as beverages until you add it up. Depending on your beverage choices, you can be adding as much as 500 to 600 extra calories per day. Fruit juices, drinking your coffee with cream or sugar, and enjoying full-fat milk are all habits you should change immediately when eating clean. Always pick water first, then herbal teas, either cold or hot, when you are thirsty.

12. **Consider your unique needs.** Clean Eating is not a one-size-fits-all plan. It is flexible enough to include any diet factor or health concern, so you should also consider your unique circumstances when planning your Clean Eating journey. If you don't look at you own needs, the whole diet strategy will fail because you will not be able to stick with it. For example, if you are an athlete, your carbohydrate intake might need to be higher than someone who is just starting to exercise.

13. **Keep track of your goals and successes.** Every diet plan encourages keeping a food journal, and this is a very good plan to keep on track. You don't have to write pages and pages of food descriptions, physical reactions, and inspirational quotes, unless you want to record these thoughts. Try keeping a small book or even a phone app where you can write your weight or health goals. This written record keeps you accountable to the reason you are eating clean, and it focuses you on long-term changes rather than just fitting into your jeans by the weekend.

14. **Add meatless Mondays to your week.** The actual meatless day doesn't matter as much as that you start incorporating vegetarian meals into your weekly routine because they are healthy and usually embody the Clean Eating priorities. If you are a hardcore carnivore, it might be a good idea to make a favorite dish such as chili with vegetarian ingredients or a simple stir-fry. Eventually a couple vegetarian meals a week is a wonderful way to get all the benefits of wholesome foods, such as produce and grains.

15. **Start cooking clean.** One of the easiest methods of getting the benefit of Clean Eating is to make sure your food preparation and cooking techniques aren't sabotaging your efforts. Watch the amount of oil you use when sautéing or use nonstick pans with water or stock instead of butter and tablespoons of vegetable oil. Make sure you lighten up on breading, bake instead of fry, and use half the dressing you usually use on salads or sandwiches. Cooking clean will allow you to taste the unique flavors of fresh foods as well, so you can gain a new appreciation for your ingredients and the combinations of herbs, spices, and other seasonings.

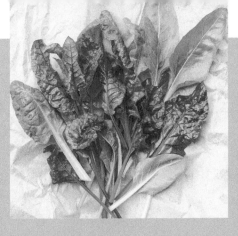

PART **TWO**

Clean Eating Recipes

Recipe Key

Selecting Recipes for Your Clean Eating Plan

The recipes in part 2 come with a great deal of additional information to help you pick and choose what foods you wish to include in your clean eating plan. Each recipe contains labels indicating what special diets it is suitable for, plus nutritional information and handy tips.

Special Diet Labels

The recipes in this book clearly indicate when they are appropriate for certain diets. You can quickly glance at a recipe and get this information right in the beginning without having to search through all the ingredients. We use the following special diet labels:

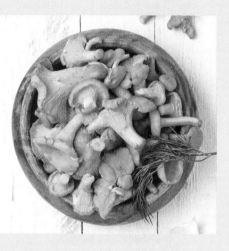

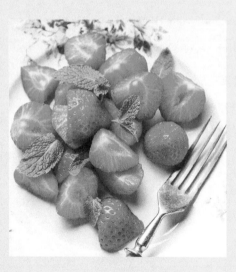

FODMAP-free: This may be a diet you are unfamiliar with if you do not suffer from Crohn's disease, irritable bowel syndrome, or colitis. It is designed to provide relief from the unpleasant symptoms associated with these conditions, such as abdominal pain, bloating, bowel changes, and gas. This diet came about when studies showed that some types of carbohydrates caused irritation in the bowels, which creates these symptoms. The carbohydrates that affect the bowels are called fermentable oligosaccharides, disaccharides, monosaccharides, and polyols, known by the acronym FODMAP. The range of foods that are not allowed on this diet include:

- Some fruits
- Some vegetables, including all alliums (such as onions, garlic, and chives)
- Grains and cereals
- Some nuts
- Sugars and other sweeteners
- Prebiotic foods
- Some alcohols
- Dairy foods

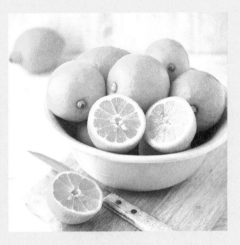

Gluten-free: This diet is often prescribed to treat celiac disease. Celiac disease affects the digestive system and can damage the small intestine, which hinders the absorption of nutrients from food. Those who suffer from this condition cannot eat gluten, a protein in wheat, barley, and rye. Avoiding gluten in all its forms can help people with celiac disease control and minimize their uncomfortable symptoms. Foods that are allowed on a gluten-free diet include:

- Some grains, such as corn, rice, and soy
- Nuts
- Seeds such as quinoa, sesame, and sunflower
- Beans
- Most dairy products
- Fresh meats, fish, eggs, and poultry
- Fruits and vegetables
- Any product specifically labeled as gluten-free

Low-fat: A great deal of research in the past few decades has pinpointed high fat consumption to an increased risk of diseases such as cardiovascular disease, obesity, and cancer. A low-fat diet decreases the likelihood of developing these conditions and many others, while supporting weight loss. Simply stated, a low-fat diet is any diet that includes no more than 30 percent of total calories as fat, and saturated fat should be no more than 10 percent. Most attention is paid to saturated fats and trans fats, which are not healthy, as opposed to monounsaturated and polyunsaturated fats, which are healthy. Foods to be avoided include red meat and whole-fat dairy products. Allowed foods include fruits, vegetables, healthy whole grains, low-fat dairy products, and lean poultry.

Low-sodium: A low-sodium diet includes no more than 1,500 mg to 2,400 mg of sodium per day. Your body needs some sodium to function efficiently, but an excess of sodium can lead to health problems such as high blood pressure, heart disease, and kidney disease. Sodium is found naturally in many foods, especially meats and fish, but it is also added through processing, cooking, and at the table via the saltshaker. If you are a healthy young adult, you can eat up to 2,300 mg of salt a day with no problems, but you should consume no more than 1,500 mg a day if:

- are fifty-one or older
- have high blood pressure, kidney disease, heart disease, or diabetes
- are African-American

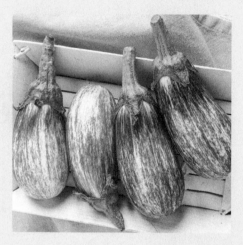

Nightshade-free: Some people have a genetic intolerance to a group of vegetables in the Solanaceae family of plants, known collectively as nightshades. These vegetables naturally produce alkaloids and saponins to protect themselves from the ravages of insects, and these substances are poisonous in large amounts. People who are sensitive to nightshade vegetables can experience gastrointestinal problems (leaky gut, bloating, nausea, and diarrhea), aching or arthritic joints, headaches, and absorption issues in the digestive tract leading to anemia and osteoporosis. Although cooking nightshade vegetables can lower the alkaloid levels by about 40 percent to 50 percent, a nightshade-free diet simply eliminates the vegetables themselves. Nightshade vegetables include:

- Capsicum family (bell peppers, jalapeño peppers, chili peppers, cayenne pepper)
- Tomato
- Potato
- Eggplant (aubergine)
- Tamarillo

- Goji berry
- Ground cherry
- Tomatillo

Vegan: A vegan diet excludes all animal products. This is why it is difficult to state definitively what a vegan diet contains, because fat-laden processed foods can be as vegan as organic fresh produce. There are many reasons why people might choose to follow a vegan diet, including health, environmental, and ethical concerns. There is a great deal of research pointing to the fact that a healthy, clean eating vegan diet reduces the risk of many diseases, including diabetes, obesity, heart disease, and cancer. The China Study by T. Colin Campbell and Thomas M. Campbell is a great resource outlining the research linking vegetable-based diets to improved health. A healthy, clean eating vegan diet includes vegetables, fruit, grains, healthy oils, nuts, legumes, and seeds. The vegan recipes in this book exclude:

- Animal or animal by-products (including meat, fish, shellfish, poultry, gelatin, rennet)
- Dairy (including milk, cheese, yogurt)
- Eggs
- Honey

Vegetarian: There are many types of vegetarian diets, depending on what you want to restrict and the reason you follow the diet. Plant-based diets can be a healthy lifestyle choice if a broad range of wholesome foods are consumed and unhealthy foods containing saturated fats and sugar are limited. A standard vegetarian diet excludes animal foods and animal by-products. However, many vegetarians still eat eggs and dairy products, and some eat fish and seafood. The recipes in this book that have the vegetarian (but not the vegan) label assume a lacto-ovo approach to diet. This means they include dairy products, eggs, and honey but do not include meat, fish, or seafood.

Nutritional Value per Serving

Calories: This is the fuel found in food that powers your body. Calories are essential for providing energy. The amount required by the body varies from person to person, depending on the individual's metabolism and activity level. If you are not an athlete or following a vigorous exercise routine, you will need between 1,600 and 2,200 calories a day to function effectively. Clean eating is not about calorie counting, but if you are trying to lose weight, you will need to eat fewer calories than you burn. If you eat an assortment of high-quality, nutritious foods and avoid processed foods, saturated fat, and sugar, you should naturally take in the right amount

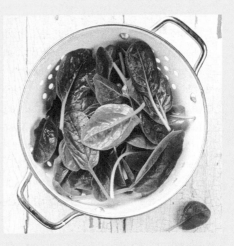

of calories. The recipes in this book assume you are following a 2,000-calorie-per-day meal plan.

Calories from fat: All calories are not created equal. This number simply reflects the calories from the fat in the dish. Do not get hung up on this piece of information unless you are on a low-fat diet, because many nutrient-packed clean eating ingredients contain a fair amount of fat. Keep in mind that this number reflects the total fat in the dish, including healthy fats that the body needs to produce hormones and absorb vitamins.

Total fat: In a healthy diet, such as a clean eating diet, you should be getting about 20 percent to 35 percent of your calories from fat. This total fat number includes all types of fat in the recipe—saturated fat, trans fat, monounsaturated fats, and polyunsaturated fats (which include omega-3 and omega-6 fatty acids). A high total-fat number can be a cause for concern, but only if it is accompanied by high saturated-fat and trans-fat percentages as well.

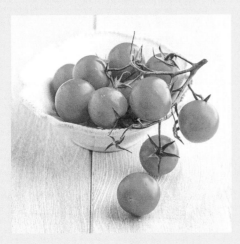

Saturated fat: Generally speaking, saturated fats are unhealthy fats—although coconut oil is an exception and can be part of a healthy diet in moderation. Saturated fats are usually animal fats. They are solid at room temperature (imagine a big, greasy brick of lard). Consuming too much saturated fat has been linked to cancer, obesity, heart disease, and other diseases. The clean eating diet recommends getting less than 10 percent of your daily calories from saturated fat.

Trans fat: This may be the most unhealthy type of fat found in food because it rarely occurs naturally—only in small amounts in some red meats and dairy products. Most trans fats are created in food production when hydrogen is added to liquid vegetable oil to make it solid. Trans fat should be almost nonexistent in a clean eating diet because it is mostly found in processed foods that are avoided on this diet. Trans fats increase the risk of heart disease, diabetes, and stroke and raise cholesterol levels. This fat should be consumed as little as possible, which is why there is no maximum

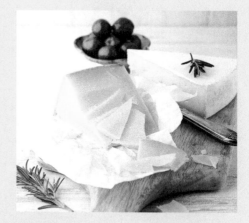

percentage of daily calories from trans fat on a clean eating list.

Sodium: When following a clean eating diet, you should try to stay under 2,300 mg of sodium a day. This basically means following a low-sodium diet. Too much sodium can create serious health problems, but clean eating plans recognize that sea salt can be a healthy part of the diet if consumed in moderation. Also remember that the sodium information in a recipe reflects one meal in a daily total. If, for example, you want to have crab for lunch, which is naturally high in sodium, balance it out with a sodium-free salad for dinner. When it comes to salt, it is the daily total that is important.

Carbs: This number shows the amount of total carbohydrates in the recipe, including fiber, starch, and sugar. The fiber in food is the indigestible part of complex carbohydrates that is found in plant foods. It is very beneficial for the digestive system and can help reduce your risk of heart disease and type 2 diabetes. Fiber does not increase blood sugar or provide energy.

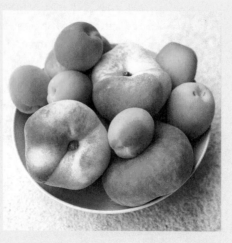

Sugar: This number shows both naturally occurring sugars and added sugars in the recipe. Refined white sugar is on the list of foods to avoid when eating clean, and you will not find that ingredient in any recipe in this book. Honey, maple syrup, and molasses, along with fruits and some vegetables, make up the majority of sugar grams in the recipes. Natural sweeteners are allowed in moderation when eating clean, but there is no set guideline for recommended grams of sugar per day.

Protein: This macronutrient is present in every cell and organ in the body and needs to be replenished daily from the food you eat. It is recommended that 10 to 35 percent of your daily calories come from protein; the amount will vary depending on your age and gender. The clean eating diet does not have a threshold number of protein grams per day, but rather advises a varied whole-food diet to ensure you don't get too much or too little protein.

Recipe Tips

These tips and insights are designed to give you more information about each recipe. You might learn an interesting preparation technique, handy shopping advice, or even how to convert a recipe to another type of diet, such as vegan or gluten-free.

- **Cooking tip:** These hints and tips will help you effectively prepare your recipes, provide advice about storage, or suggest interesting cooking techniques or shortcuts.

- **Diet tip:** The information found here will help you change the ingredients or technique in the recipe to create a dish that follows one of the special diets listed previously in this section.

- **Leftovers tip:** What happens if you use only half of an ingredient in a recipe or have leftovers from your meal? This tip will give you ideas about how to use up the ingredient or create a new dish the next day using the leftovers.

- **Nutrition tip:** You will find specific health benefits and unique characteristics of certain ingredients in the recipe here.

- **Shopping tip:** These are tips about the best seasons to buy specific foods, what to look for to get the best ingredients, and ideas on how to save money on more expensive ingredients.

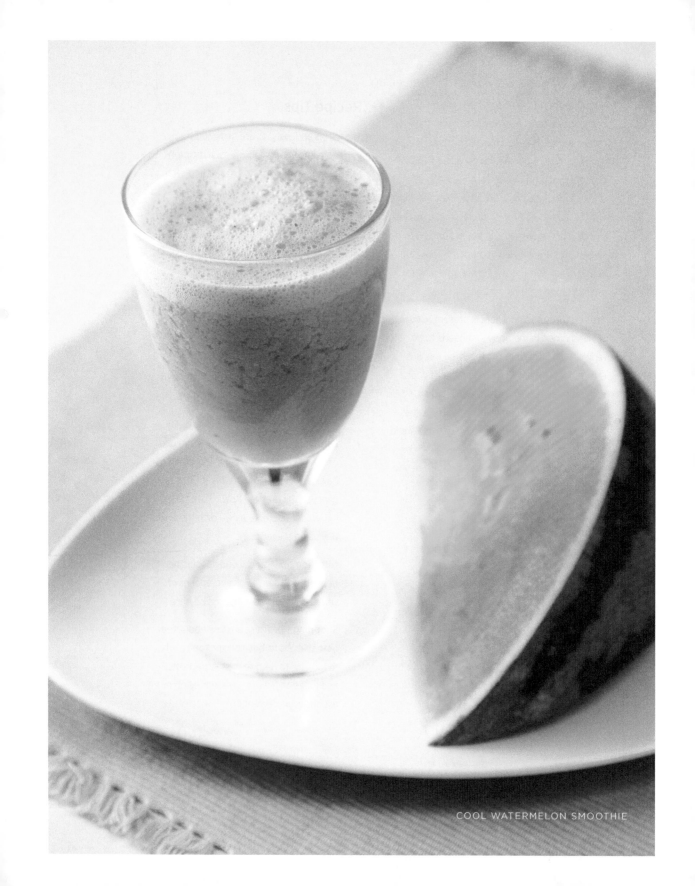

COOL WATERMELON SMOOTHIE

CHAPTER FOUR

CHAPTER FOUR

Smoothies

Gluten-free
Low-fat
Low-sodium
Nightshade-free
Vegetarian

SMOOTHIES

Green Tea, Blackberry, and Banana Smoothie

Green tea might not be the first ingredient you think of when making a smoothie, but it can be a delicious, healthy choice to combine with your favorite fruits or vegetables. Green tea has been used as a medicinal drink in Asia for centuries and is linked to improving or preventing many health problems, such as high blood pressure, diabetes, and cancer. Green tea is not processed, like black teas, so it contains powerful antioxidants.

Cooking tip If you want to make green tea a regular ingredient in your smoothies, you can steep a large batch of tea and keep it in your refrigerator in a sealed container for easy use.

⅓ cup hot water (not boiling)

1 green tea bag

2 tablespoons honey

3 cups fresh blackberries

1 medium banana

2 cups vanilla almond milk

3 cups ice cubes

1. In a small bowl, pour the water over the tea bag.
2. Steep the tea for about 4 minutes and then remove the tea bag.
3. Stir the honey into the tea and put the tea in the refrigerator until cool, about 20 minutes.
4. In a blender, combine the blackberries, banana, and vanilla almond milk and pulse until smooth.
5. Add the tea and the ice cubes and blend until the drink is smooth.
6. Pour into glasses and serve.

Serves 2. Prep time 7 minutes.

Calories **239** / Calories from fat **32** / Total fat **3.6g** / Saturated fat **0.0g** / Trans fat **0.0g** / Sodium **164mg** / Carbs **52.5g** / Sugars **34.8g** / Protein **4.6g**

Papaya Yogurt Smoothie

Gluten-free
Low-fat
Low-sodium
Nightshade-free
Vegetarian

SMOOTHIES

This smoothie is a lovely pastel pink and is packed with flavor and energy-boosting ingredients. If you are looking for relief from sports injuries or other aches and pains, the enzyme found in papaya—papain—and the enzyme in pineapple—bromelain—are effective treatments. Papaya is also heart-friendly and can help prevent atherosclerosis.

Shopping tip Ripe papayas are slightly soft to the touch and have orange skin. The antioxidant level of the fruit increases as the fruit ripens. Store ripe papayas in the refrigerator and eat them within two or three days.

2 medium papayas, peeled, seeded, and cut into chunks

2 cups Greek yogurt

1 cup fresh pineapple, peeled, cored, and cut into chunks

1 tablespoon pure vanilla extract

3 cups ice cubes

1. In a blender, combine all the ingredients except the ice and pulse until smooth.
2. Add the ice cubes and blend until smooth.
3. Pour into glasses and serve.

Serves 2. Prep time 6 minutes.

Calories **384** / Calories from fat **90** / Total fat **10.0g** / Saturated fat **6.2g** / Trans fat **0.0g** / Sodium **113mg** / Carbs **54.7g** / Sugars **42.5g** / Protein **22.0g**

Gluten-free
Low-fat
Low-sodium
Nightshade-free
Vegetarian

SMOOTHIES

Cool Watermelon Smoothie

Summer in a glass is the best description of this tasty treat. Watermelon is extremely high in antioxidants, especially lycopene, which is wonderful for the cardiovascular system. It can help improve blood flow, which can reduce blood pressure. Watermelon is also a good source of iron and zinc, which are minerals that support a healthy heart.

Nutrition tip Watermelon has the highest amount of antioxidants when ripe and juicy red. Once a watermelon is ripe, the antioxidant levels stay stable for about two days. Choose red watermelons rather than yellow if you want the greatest lycopene benefits.

4 cups chopped watermelon

½ cup unsweetened apple juice

4 cups ice cubes

1. In a blender, combine the watermelon and apple juice and pulse until blended, about 30 seconds.
2. Add the ice cubes and blend until smooth, about 30 seconds.
3. Pour into glasses and serve immediately.

Serves 2. Prep time 4 minutes.

Calories **112** / Calories from fat **5** / Total fat **0.5g** / Saturated fat **0.0g** / Trans fat: **0.0g** / Sodium **29mg** / Carbs **30.2g** / Sugars **22.0g** / Protein **3.9g**

Oatmeal–Peanut Butter Smoothie

If you have a busy day planned, peanut butter is the perfect food to boost your energy and help you feel full longer. Peanut butter has many nutrients such as protein, potassium, fiber, and healthy fat. It is also a good source of magnesium and vitamin E.

Shopping tip Try to buy natural peanut butter. The fat content of most peanut butters is the same regardless of whether it is processed, but natural products contain only healthy fats, while processed peanut butter can have other unhealthy fats added.

1 large banana

½ cup rolled oats

½ cup Greek yogurt

½ cup skim milk

2 tablespoons natural peanut butter

2 cups ice cubes

1. In a blender, combine the banana, oats, yogurt, milk, and peanut butter, and blend until smooth.
2. Add the ice cubes and blend until smooth.
3. Pour into glasses and serve.

Serves 2. Prep time 5 minutes.

Calories **336** / Calories from fat **102** / Total fat **11.3g** / Saturated fat **3.3g** / Trans fat: **0.0g** / Sodium **77mg** / Carbs **39.3g** / Sugars **16.3g** / Protein **20.4g**

Creamy Orange Smoothie

Oranges are one of the most popular fruits because they are so sweet and have a glorious, cheerful color. This smoothie, with the combination of mango and orange, is like sunshine in a glass. Oranges help prevent several types of cancer, improve heart health, and promote good vision.

Cooking tip If you want your drink to be smooth and silky, you can segment your orange before putting it in a blender rather than leaving all the membranes intact. Simply peel the orange using a sharp paring knife to cut away the pith as well as the peel. Then cut the segments out of the orange by following the membranes.

1 cup plain Greek yogurt

1 cup almond milk

1 large mango, peeled and cut into chunks

1 large orange, peeled and chopped into chunks

1 teaspoon pure vanilla extract

2 cups ice cubes

1. In a blender, combine the yogurt, almond milk, mango, orange, and vanilla and pulse until smooth.
2. Add the ice cubes and blend until smooth.
3. Pour into glasses and serve.

Serves 2. Prep time 5 minutes.

Calories **237** / Calories from fat **60** / Total fat **6.6g** / Saturated fat **3.2g** / Trans fat **0.0g** / Sodium **130mg** / Carbs **34.2g** / Sugars **28.9g** / Protein **11.9g**

Kiwi Mint Smoothie

Gluten-free
Low-fat
Low-sodium
Nightshade-free
Vegan
Vegetarian

SMOOTHIES

The cool, minty goodness of this smoothie might remind you of a breeze-kissed veranda in the South. Kiwi is one of the safest fruits to consume if you do not buy organic. For several years it has been on the list of produce that is least contaminated with pesticides. You can also use golden kiwi in this recipe, but the smoothie might not be as green.

Cooking tip If you have a nice big bunch of fresh mint and don't use it all in one recipe, try puréeing the mint and freezing the purée in ice cube trays. For this smoothie, add one frozen mint cube instead of using fresh leaves.

2 large kiwis, peeled and cut into slices

2 cups fresh pineapple, peeled, cored, and cut into chunks

1 cup almond milk

15 fresh mint leaves

1 cup ice cubes

1. In a blender, combine the kiwis, pineapple, almond milk, and mint, and pulse until smooth.
2. Add the ice and blend until the drink is well mixed and smooth.
3. Pour into glasses and serve.

Serves 2. Prep time 4 minutes.

Calories **172** / Calories from fat **18** / Total fat **2.0g** / Saturated fat **0.0g** / Trans fat **0.0g** / Sodium **78mg** / Carbs **40.4g** / Sugars **27.4g** / Protein **2.8g**

FODMAP-free
Gluten-free
Low-fat
Low-sodium
Nightshade-free
Vegan
Vegetarian

SMOOTHIES

Cucumber Ginger Smoothie

Several ingredients in this refreshing drink are beneficial to the digestive system. It is great for improving an upset stomach or even as part of a healthy detox plan. Ginger soothes the intestines, eliminates gas, and can relieve the symptoms of motion or morning sickness.

Nutrition tip Cucumbers have a high water and fiber content, which can assist the digestive process. They can help clear toxins from the body, and, as part of a daily meal plan, can improve heartburn, gastritis, and ulcers.

1 large English cucumber, washed and cut into chunks

1 teaspoon grated fresh ginger

1 cup water, plus more if necessary

Juice of ½ large lemon

¼ cup mint leaves

1 cup ice cubes

1. In a blender, combine the cucumber, ginger, water, lemon juice, and mint. Blend until smooth.
2. Add the ice and blend until smooth, adding more water if the smoothie is too thick.
3. Pour into glasses and serve.

Serves 2. Prep time 5 minutes.

Calories **35** / Calories from fat **5** / Total fat **0.5g** / Saturated fat **0.0g** / Trans fat **0.0g** / Sodium **10mg** / Carbs **7.1g** / Sugar **0.0g** / Protein **1.4g**

Green Strawberry Smoothie

SMOOTHIES

This refreshing smoothie has all the goodness of spinach, with a surprising strawberry taste. The texture is not completely smooth because of the strawberry seeds, but the seeds are a rich source of fiber so are a healthy addition to the smoothie.

Cooking tip You can use fresh strawberries for this smoothie for a more intense berry taste. If you use fresh berries, you have to add an extra cup of ice or use a frozen banana to get the right thick texture.

1½ cups unsweetened almond milk

2 cups packed baby spinach greens

1 cup frozen unsweetened strawberries

1 banana

1 cup ice

1. Place the almond milk, spinach, strawberries, and banana in a blender and purée until smooth.
2. Add the ice and blend until the smoothie is a milkshake consistency. Pour the smoothie into 2 glasses to serve.

Serves 2. Prep time 10 minutes.

Calories **107** / Calories from fat **18** / Total fat **2.0g** / Saturated fat **0.0g** / Sodium **159mg** / Carbs **21.8g** / Sugars **11.6g** / Protein **2.2g**

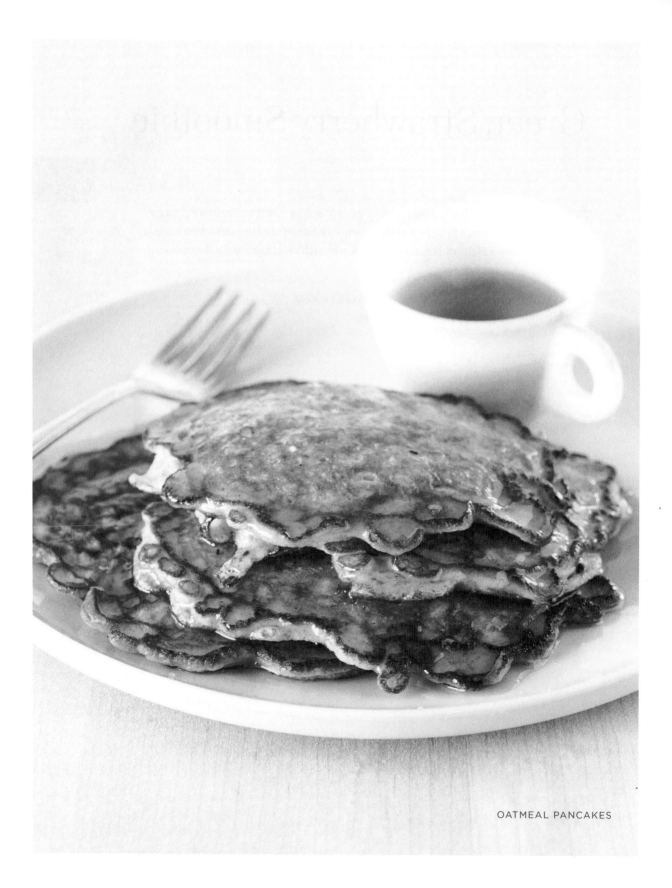

OATMEAL PANCAKES

CHAPTER FIVE

Breakfast

Oatmeal Chia Breakfast Pudding

You will love the convenience of this creamy porridge because there is no cooking involved, and it can be made the night before. Chia seeds can absorb about ten times their volume, so make sure you use enough liquid in your preparation. Chia supports healthy weight-loss goals, can help stabilize blood sugar, and promotes an efficient digestive system.

Diet tip If you want to create a gluten-free dish, buy gluten-free oats instead of regular ones. Chia seeds are already gluten-free.

1½ cups vanilla almond milk

¼ cup chia seeds

¼ cup rolled oats

¼ cup honey

1 teaspoon ground cinnamon

1 teaspoon pure vanilla extract

1 large banana, peeled and sliced

½ cup sliced strawberries

1. In a medium bowl, stir together the almond milk, chia seeds, oats, honey, cinnamon, and vanilla until very well combined.
2. Let the mixture sit for about 15 minutes in the refrigerator, until the liquid is absorbed.
3. Serve topped with sliced banana and strawberries.

Serves 2. Prep time 15 minutes.

Calories **395** / Calories from fat **119** / Total fat **13.3g** / Saturated fat **1.0g** / Trans fat **0.0g** / Sodium **138mg** / Carbs **67.4g** / Sugars **46.0g** / Protein **9.3g**

Coconut Quinoa Porridge

Quinoa is an ancient grain that fits right into the clean eating diet. Although cooked like a grain, this tasty food is actually a seed, making it gluten-free. Quinoa is a complete protein, which means it contains the nine essential amino acids that the body does not produce. There are more than one hundred varieties of quinoa, but you will probably find only the white, red, and black types in your local grocery store.

Cooking tip Always wash your quinoa thoroughly. It is coated with saponins, which have a slightly bitter, soapy taste. Some people are sensitive to this substance, which makes this step a must.

¼ teaspoon extra-virgin coconut oil

1 teaspoon ground cinnamon

½ cup quinoa, rinsed

½ cup almond milk

½ cup light coconut milk

1 teaspoon honey

1 tablespoon unsweetened
   shredded coconut

1 cup blueberries

1. In a medium saucepan over medium-high heat, heat the oil and cinnamon for about 1 minute.
2. Add the quinoa and stir until coated with the oil.
3. Stir in the almond milk and coconut milk and bring the mixture to a boil.
4. Reduce the heat to low so the mixture simmers and then cover the saucepan.
5. Continue to simmer until the quinoa has absorbed all the milk, about 10 minutes.
6. Stir in the honey.
7. Serve topped with coconut and blueberries.

Serves 2. Prep time 10 minutes. Cook time 15 minutes.

Calories **247** / Calories from fat **38** / Total fat **4.2g** / Saturated fat **1.1g** / Trans fat **0.0g** / Sodium **64mg** / Carbs **37.8g** / Sugars **14.9g** / Protein **8.7g**

Sunny Corn Cakes

They are less dense than traditional cornbread and are best if you use fresh corn taken right off the cob. You can leave out the maple syrup if you are watching your sweetener intake; these cakes will still be just as tasty without it.

Diet tip This recipe can be vegan if you exclude the yogurt. These cakes are delicious even without the creamy topping.

½ cup vanilla almond milk

½ teaspoon apple cider vinegar

¼ cup yellow cornmeal

¼ cup whole-wheat pastry flour

1 teaspoon baking powder

Pinch of sea salt

Pinch of ground nutmeg

2 tablespoons pure maple syrup

1 tablespoon olive oil

½ cup fresh or frozen corn kernels

Nonstick cooking spray

4 tablespoons Greek yogurt

1. In a medium bowl, whisk together the almond milk and vinegar and set aside for 5 minutes to thicken.
2. In a small bowl, combine the cornmeal, flour, baking powder, salt, and nutmeg and set aside.
3. Add the maple syrup and olive oil to the almond milk mixture and stir to combine.
4. Add the dry ingredients and the corn into the milk mixture and stir until just combined.
5. Put the batter in the refrigerator for about 10 minutes.
6. In a large skillet over medium-high heat, add a light coat of cooking spray.
7. Add the batter, 3 tablespoons per cake, and cook until bubbles form, about 2 minutes. Flip the cakes over and cook the other side until golden, about 1 minute.
8. Transfer to a plate and repeat with remaining batter.
9. Serve three cakes per portion, topped with 1 tablespoon of yogurt.

Serves 4. Prep time 15 minutes. Cook time 15 minutes.

Calories **155** / Calories from fat **46** / Total fat **5.1g** / Saturated fat **1.0g** / Trans fat **0.0g** / Sodium **94mg** / Carbs **24.4g** / Sugars **7.8g** / Protein **4.6g**

Apricot Cranberry Breakfast Bars

Low-fat
Low-sodium
Nightshade-free
Vegetarian

BREAKFAST

Once you try homemade granola bars, you will never buy the packaged, processed version again. You can use any dried fruit or nuts in these bars, such as raisins, dried blueberries or cherries, pecans, and cashews for interesting variations.

Cooking tip These bars freeze very well, so make a double batch and keep some stored for a quick grab-and-go breakfast or even a snack throughout the day.

Olive oil cooking spray

4 cups rolled oats

1 cup whole-wheat flour

½ teaspoon ground nutmeg

½ teaspoon ground cinnamon

4 egg whites

1 cup unsweetened applesauce

¼ cup honey

1 teaspoon pure vanilla extract

½ cup chopped dried apricots

½ cup dried cranberries

4 tablespoons slivered almonds

1. Preheat the oven to 350°F. Lightly coat a 12-by-8-inch baking dish with cooking spray and set aside.
2. In a medium bowl, stir together the oats, flour, nutmeg, and cinnamon. Mix well.
3. In a large bowl, whisk together the egg whites, applesauce, honey, and vanilla until well blended.
4. Add the oat mixture to the wet ingredients and stir to combine.
5. Stir in the apricots, cranberries, and almonds.
6. Spoon the mixture into the baking dish, smoothing out the top.
7. Bake for 20 to 25 minutes, or until a toothpick inserted in the center comes out clean.
8. Let the uncut bars cool on a wire rack until they reach room temperature. Cut into 16 bars and store in a sealed container in the refrigerator or freezer.

Makes 16 bars. Prep time 15 minutes. Cook time 25 minutes.

Calories **146** / Calories from fat **20** / Total fat **2.2g** / Saturated fat **0.0g** / Trans fat **0.0g** / Sodium **16mg** / Carbs **27.3g** / Sugars **6.8g** / Protein **4.8g**

Oatmeal Pancakes

You would never know these pretty golden pancakes have cottage cheese in them as a base. Although technically it's not clean, cottage cheese is an excellent source of protein, calcium, vitamin B_{12}, and phosphorus. The extra fiber from the oatmeal makes this an incredibly nutritious start to the day.

Tasty Tip The vanilla extract adds a lovely sweet taste to these pancakes, but you can substitute almond extract for a satisfying nutty taste. If you opt for almond extract, sprinkle some slivered almonds on the pancakes to double up on the flavor.

3 egg whites

½ cup low-fat cottage cheese

1 tablespoon pure maple syrup

½ teaspoon pure vanilla extract

½ teaspoon ground cinnamon

½ cup rolled oats

Nonstick cooking spray

1. In a food processor combine the egg whites, cottage cheese, maple syrup, vanilla, and cinnamon and pulse until very well blended, about 1 minute.
2. Add the oatmeal and pulse for an additional 30 seconds.
3. In a large skillet over medium heat, add a light coat of cooking spray.
4. Pour about ¼ cup of batter onto the skillet for each pancake; do not overcrowd.
5. Cook until the tops of the pancakes start to bubble and then flip the pancakes over.
6. Cook for an additional minute until the pancakes are cooked through and golden brown.
7. Repeat until all the batter is used up.
8. Serve 3 pancakes, warm or cold, per person.

Makes 2 servings. Prep time 2 minutes. Cook time 15 minutes.

Calories **185** / Calories from fat **26** / Total fat **2.9g** / Saturated fat **1.0g** / Trans fat **0.0g** / Sodium **314mg** / Carbs **23.5g** / Sugars **6.8g** / Protein **15.9g**

Simple Potato Frittata

Gluten-free
Low-fat
Vegetarian

BREAKFAST

Potatoes have a bad reputation with healthy eaters, but they are actually very nutritious. It is the deep frying of French fries and the fatty toppings on baked potatoes, such as sour cream and butter, that make them seem bad. Potatoes in their clean form are packed with fiber and low in calories.

Leftovers tip Frittatas are just as delicious cold. Cut your leftover frittata into portions and store them individually for a quick snack, light lunch, or a no-hassle breakfast the next day.

10 new potatoes, washed and cut
    into quarters

1 egg

6 egg whites

3 teaspoons skim milk

3 tablespoons finely chopped fresh parsley

1 tablespoon chopped fresh rosemary

Pinch of freshly ground black pepper

Pinch of sea salt

1 teaspoon olive oil

1 small sweet onion, peeled and diced

1 teaspoon minced garlic

1. In a medium saucepan, cover the potatoes with water by about 1 inch and bring to a boil over medium-high heat.
2. Reduce the heat to low, and simmer until the potatoes are tender, about 10 minutes.
3. Drain the potatoes and set aside.
4. In a medium bowl, whisk together the egg, egg whites, milk, parsley, rosemary, pepper, and salt.
5. In a medium skillet over medium-high heat, heat the oil and sauté the onion until it is tender and lightly browned, about 5 minutes.
6. Add the garlic and sauté for an additional minute.
7. Add the cooked potatoes to the skillet and stir to combine.
8. Pour the egg mixture into the skillet, shaking the pan gently to distribute the egg evenly.
9. Cover the skillet and cook until the eggs are just set, about 10 minutes.

continued ➤

Simple Potato Frittata *continued*

10. Remove the skillet from the heat and let the frittata sit for about 15 minutes.
11. Cut the finished frittata into 4 wedges and serve.

Serves 4. Prep time 10 minutes. Cook time 35 minutes.

Calories **271** / Calories from fat **26** / Total fat **2.9g** / Saturated fat **0.7g** / Trans fat **0.0g** / Sodium **121mg** / Carbs **36.7g** / Sugars **4.8g** / Protein **12.4g** /

Poached Eggs
over Sweet Potatoes

This is a truly lovely dish that is simple to put together and makes a meal for a large gathering, if you double or triple the recipe. Don't worry if the yolks on the eggs break; they will simply run into the hash underneath and the dish will still taste delicious.

Diet tip The sunny, rich yolks of these poached eggs are an important part of a healthy diet because they contain essential fatty acids and vitamins. Yolks are beneficial to the heart because they can help reduce homocysteine in the liver, which is a compound that can increase the risk of heart disease.

1 teaspoon olive oil

2 medium sweet potatoes, peeled and
   diced into ½-inch pieces

½ small sweet onion, peeled and diced into
   ½-inch pieces

¼ teaspoon ground cumin

¼ teaspoon smoked paprika

Pinch of sea salt

Pinch of freshly ground black pepper

2 tablespoons finely chopped fresh parsley

1 teaspoon white vinegar

2 eggs

1. In a large skillet over medium heat, heat the olive oil and sauté the sweet potatoes and onions, stirring frequently, for about 15 minutes or until the potatoes are tender.
2. Add the cumin, paprika, salt, and pepper. Continue sautéing until the potatoes are browned, about 5 minutes.
3. Stir in the parsley and sauté for 1 minute more.
4. Set the skillet aside, covered.
5. Meanwhile, in a large saucepan over high heat, boil 4 to 5 inches of water.
6. Stir in the vinegar, and bring to a boil again.
7. Reduce the heat to low, so the water is gently simmering.
8. Crack one egg into a small bowl.

continued ➤

Poached Eggs over Sweet Potatoes *continued*

9. Gently slip the egg into the simmering water and repeat with the other egg.
10. Poach the eggs for about 3 minutes, or until the whites are firm.
11. Remove the poached eggs with a slotted spoon and drain them on paper towels.
12. Spoon the sweet potato hash onto two plates and top each portion with a poached egg.

Serves 2. Prep time 5 minutes. Cook time 25 minutes.

Calories **280** / Calories from fat **69** / Total fat **7.7g** / Saturated fat **2.0g** / Trans fat **0.0g** / Sodium **86mg** / Carbs **44.4g** / Sugars **2.0g** / Protein **8.9g** /

Vegetable Hash

Gluten-free
Low-fat
Low-sodium
Vegan
Vegetarian

BREAKFAST

The broccoli elevates this hash into super-food territory. This vegetable may help prevent many types of cancer and detoxify the body. Broccoli is an excellent source of vitamins K, C, and A, plus fiber and chromium. It is also very low on the glycemic index, which means eating plenty of this vegetable can decrease your risk of kidney disease, type 2 diabetes, and cardiovascular disease.

Cooking tip To save time, roast the squash and potatoes the day before and then sauté them along with the onion and broccoli to warm them up.

½ small butternut squash, peeled and cut into ½-inch chunks

10 small new potatoes, quartered

1 teaspoon chopped fresh thyme

¼ teaspoon sea salt

¼ teaspoon freshly ground black pepper

2 teaspoons olive oil, divided

½ small sweet onion, peeled and diced

1 head broccoli, cut into small florets

1 small red bell pepper, seeded and cut into thin strips

1 teaspoon fresh lemon juice

1 teaspoon chopped fresh parsley

1. Preheat the oven to 425°F. Line a baking sheet with foil and set aside.
2. In a large bowl, toss the squash and potatoes together with the thyme, salt, pepper, and 1 teaspoon of the oil until well combined.
3. Transfer the squash and potatoes to the baking sheet and bake, stirring occasionally, until the vegetables are tender, about 20 minutes.
4. Remove the squash and potatoes from the oven and set aside.
5. In a large skillet over medium-high heat, heat the remaining 1 teaspoon of olive oil and sauté the onion and broccoli until tender, about 5 minutes.
6. Add the red pepper and sauté for an additional minute.
7. Add the squash and potatoes to the skillet along with the lemon juice and parsley, and stir until heated through and well mixed, about 5 minutes.
8. Serve warm.

Serves 6. Prep time 5 minutes. Cook time 35 minutes.

Calories **194** / Calories from fat **17** / Total fat **1.9g** / Saturated fat **0.0g** / Trans fat **0.0g** / Sodium **98mg** / Carbs **21.3g** / Sugars **4.8g** / Protein **4.7g**

Turkey Sausage Patties

Sausage can be a lovely, lean addition to any breakfast if you make your own and use extra-lean turkey breast as a base. This sausage has a definite fiery kick to it, with lots of ginger and fresh jalapeño pepper. If you want to reduce the heat, simply decrease the quantities of these ingredients.

Diet tip If you are trying to avoid nightshade vegetables, omit the jalapeño pepper from your ingredients.

1 pound extra-lean ground turkey breast
1 small apple, peeled, cored, and
    diced small
2 large green onions, chopped finely
1 fresh jalapeño pepper, seeded and
    chopped finely

1 tablespoon grated fresh ginger
1 tablespoon chopped fresh cilantro
Pinch of sea salt
Pinch of freshly ground black pepper
1 tablespoon olive oil

1. In a medium bowl, combine all the ingredients except the oil until very well mixed.
2. Form the sausage mixture into 8 patties, each about 3 inches in diameter.
3. In a large skillet over medium heat, heat the oil and cook the patties until golden and completely cooked through, about 4 minutes per side.
4. Serve 2 patties per person with greens or a hardboiled egg.

Serves 4. Prep time 5 minutes. Cook time 10 minutes.

Calories **179** / Calories from fat **42** / Total fat **4.6g** / Saturated fat **0.5g** / Trans fat **0.0g** / Sodium **131mg** / Carbs **7.0g** / Sugars **4.3g** / Protein **26.4g**

Eggs Baked in Ratatouille

Gluten-free
Low-sodium
Vegetarian

BREAKFAST

Ratatouille is considered to be a rustic dish, but there is an elegance to the perfect combination of textures, tastes, and colors. It is even more perfectly balanced by the rich, almost buttery baked eggs. The mix of different colored vegetables ensures you will be eating a healthy range of nutrients as well.

Cooking tip The best eggs for baking are the freshest you can find, because the whites thin out after about a week in the refrigerator. Thin whites mean your eggs will not hold together as well. This is also true for poaching eggs.

1 teaspoon olive oil

1 medium red onion, peeled and chopped

1 tablespoon minced garlic

1 red bell pepper, seeded and diced

1 yellow bell pepper, seeded and diced

1 small eggplant, diced

2 small zucchini, diced

3 large tomatoes, diced

½ cup water

2 teaspoons balsamic vinegar

1 tablespoon chopped fresh oregano

Pinch of crushed red pepper flakes

4 eggs

1. In a large skillet over medium-high heat, heat the oil and sauté the onion until tender, about 3 minutes.
2. Add the garlic and sauté for 1 minute more.
3. Add the peppers, eggplant, and zucchini and sauté for 3 minutes.
4. Add the tomatoes, water, and vinegar and stir to combine.
5. Bring the vegetable mixture to a boil.
6. Reduce the heat to low and simmer the ratatouille, uncovered, for 20 minutes.
7. Stir in the oregano and the red pepper flakes.
8. With the back of a large spoon, make four deep indents in the vegetable mixture and carefully crack an egg into each indent.
9. Cover the skillet and cook for 4 more minutes, or until the egg whites are firm.
10. Serve immediately.

Serves 4. Prep time 15 minutes. Cook time 40 minutes.

Calories **162** / Calories from fat **62** / Total fat **6.9g** / Saturated fat **1.8g** / Trans fat **0.0g** / Sodium **81mg** / Carbs **19.9g** / Sugars **9.1g** / Protein **9.4g**

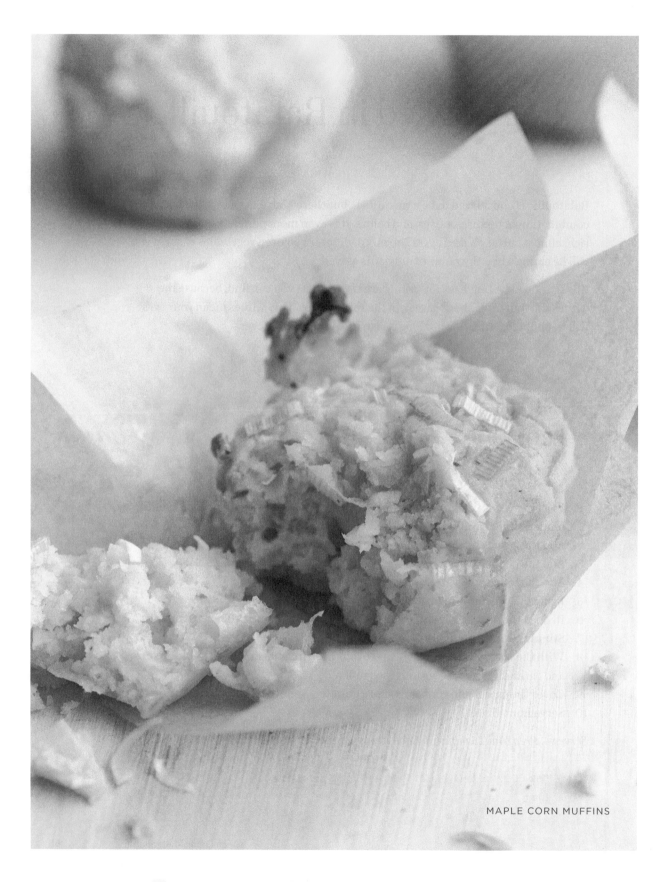

MAPLE CORN MUFFINS

Snacks

Gluten-free
Low-sodium
Nightshade-free
Vegan
Vegetarian

CHAPTER SIX

SNACKS

Garlic Roasted Chickpeas

Roasting chickpeas creates a crunchy, golden treat that makes a great grab-and-go snack for kids and adults alike. You can flavor these with any assortment of seasonings you feel will work, such as chili powder, thyme, and curry. You can also omit the savory ingredients and try cinnamon or nutmeg instead.

Cooking tip Do not skip the step of drying your chickpeas, because otherwise the oil will not coat evenly and your finished snack will not be crunchy.

3 cups canned sodium-free chickpeas, rinsed and drained

2 teaspoons olive oil

1 teaspoon minced garlic

Pinch of sea salt

Freshly ground black pepper

1. Lay out paper towels on a work surface and spread the chickpeas on the towels to dry for about 30 minutes.
2. Preheat the oven to 375°F.
3. In a large bowl, toss the dried chickpeas with the oil, garlic, salt, and pepper until well coated.
4. On a baking sheet, spread the chickpeas evenly and bake until golden and crisp, about 45 minutes.
5. Allow the chickpeas to cool completely. Store them in a sealed container at room temperature for up to 5 days.

Serves 5. Prep time 10 minutes. Cook time 45 minutes.

Calories **70** / Calories from fat **23** / Total fat **2.5g** / Saturated fat **0.0g** / Trans fat **0.0g** / Sodium **52mg** / Carbs **8.1g** / Sugar **0.0g** / Protein **3.7g**

Apple Pie Fruit Leathers

Gluten-free
Low-fat
Low-sodium
Nightshade-free
Vegan
Vegetarian

SNACKS

Fruit leathers sold in colorful packaging to kids are nothing like these flavorful apple-packed treats. The trick to great fruit leather is to spread the ingredients very thinly and evenly on the baking sheets. Try using a metal baker's spatula (also called an offset spatula) to achieve the perfect layer.

Nutrition tip Apples are one of the most nutritious foods on the planet, and eating one a day might really keep the doctor away! They are incredibly high in antioxidants that help repair the effects of free radicals and fight disease.

4 cups unsweetened applesauce

1 teaspoon ground cinnamon

½ teaspoon ground nutmeg

½ teaspoon ground ginger

Pinch of ground cloves

1. Preheat the oven to the lowest setting possible, or 140°F. Line two baking sheets with parchment paper and set aside.
2. In a medium bowl, combine all the ingredients until very well mixed.
3. Spread 2 cups of the apple mixture onto each baking sheet. Take your time, and make the layer even and thin.
4. Bake or dehydrate the mixture in the oven until it is completely dried and no longer tacky, about 6 hours.
5. Remove the baking sheets from the oven and cut the leathers into 20 pieces.
6. Store the leathers in a sealed container in the refrigerator for up to 1 week.

Makes 20 fruit leathers. Prep time 5 minutes. Cook time 6 hours.

Calories **22** / Calories from fat **0** / Total fat **0.0g** / Saturated fat **0.0g** / Trans fat **0.0g** / Sodium **1mg** / Carbs **5.7g** / Sugars **4.9g** / Protein **0.1g**

Low-fat
Low-sodium
Nightshade-free
Vegan
Vegetarian

SNACKS

Gingerbread Granola Bars

These bars have a complex, warm taste enhanced by the molasses. Gingerbread often contains molasses as a natural complement to the flavor, but molasses is also very healthy. It is a safe sweetener for diabetics because it is not high on the glycemic index. Molasses is also rich in iron, copper, calcium, and magnesium.

Cooking tip If you are a true ginger enthusiast, replace the ground ginger with 2 tablespoons of freshly grated ginger.

3 cups rolled oats

½ cup cranberries

½ cup slivered almonds

1 teaspoon ground ginger

1 teaspoon ground cinnamon

½ teaspoon ground nutmeg

¼ teaspoon baking soda

½ cup unsweetened applesauce

⅓ cup pure maple syrup

3 tablespoons molasses

1 teaspoon pure vanilla extract

1. Preheat the oven to 350°F. Line a 9-by-13-inch baking dish with parchment paper and set aside.
2. In a large bowl, combine the oats, cranberries, almonds, ginger, cinnamon, nutmeg, and baking soda.
3. In a small bowl, stir together the applesauce, maple syrup, molasses, and vanilla.
4. Add the wet ingredients to the dry ingredients and stir until mixed well.
5. Transfer the oat mixture to the baking dish, spread evenly, and press down firmly.
6. Bake for 20 minutes and then remove the dish from the oven.
7. Allow the mixture to cool for about 30 minutes and then score, but do not cut, into 16 bars.
8. Cool completely and slip the parchment paper with the scored-bars from the pan. Cut through the score marks.
9. Store the granola bars in a sealed container in the refrigerator for up to 1 week.

Makes 16 bars. Prep time 5 minutes. Cook time 20 minutes.

Calories **111** / Calories from fat **23** / Total fat **2.5g** / Saturated fat **0.7g** / Trans fat **0.0g** / Sodium **22mg** / Carbs **19.7g** / Sugars **7.2g** / Protein **2.7g**

Thai Chicken Endive Boats

Belgium endive leaves make perfect crunchy containers for all sorts of tasty fillings, and they don't add extra fat or calories to the finished dish. Endive is high in vitamin A, vitamin C, calcium, iron, potassium, and fiber. It can be slightly bitter, especially if the leaves are bigger. Try to pick the medium to small leaves for these filled boats.

Leftovers tip The endive leaves that are too big or small for this dish can be used in a salad or shredded for sandwiches and wraps.

One 6-ounce boneless, skinless cooked
    chicken breast, shredded
1 cup shredded carrots
1 cup bean sprouts
1 green onion, finely chopped
2 tablespoons chopped fresh cilantro
2 tablespoons fresh lime juice

2 teaspoons grated fresh ginger
1 tablespoon natural almond butter
1 teaspoon rice vinegar
1 teaspoon olive oil
2 large Belgium endive heads, separated
    into 12 medium leaves

1. In a medium bowl, combine the chicken, carrot, bean sprouts, green onion, cilantro, lime juice, and ginger until well mixed.
2. In a small bowl, whisk the almond butter, vinegar, and oil together to make the dressing and set aside.
3. Arrange the endive leaves on a serving plate and spoon the chicken mixture into the leaves.
4. Drizzle the stuffed endive leaves with the dressing and serve.

Makes 12 appetizers. Prep time 15 minutes.

Calories **64** / Calories from fat **22** / Total fat **2.4g** / Saturated fat **1.2g** / Trans fat **0.0g** /
Sodium **35mg** / Carbs **5.5g** / Sugars **0.9g** / Protein **6.0g**

Spiced Chicken Meatballs

This is a perfect choice for a slightly exotic casual dish for a party, although it is a bit messy to eat if you use flatbread. It can even be placed in the center of the table for a family-style meal. You can substitute lean ground turkey or pork in this dish for a different taste and texture.

Diet tip If you want a gluten-free dish, omit the flatbreads and serve the curried meatballs over quinoa or brown rice.

1 pound lean ground chicken

2 green onions, finely chopped

Pinch of sea salt

1 teaspoon olive oil

2 teaspoons grated fresh ginger

1 teaspoon ground coriander

½ teaspoon ground cumin

4 cups fat-free, low-sodium chicken stock

1 bay leaf

3 cups cauliflower florets

1 teaspoon chopped fresh cilantro

2 whole-wheat flatbreads, cut in half

1. In a medium bowl, mix together the chicken, green onions, and salt until well combined.
2. Form the chicken mixture into 12 meatballs and set aside.
3. In a large skillet over medium-high heat, heat the oil and sauté the ginger, coriander, and cumin until fragrant, about 1 minute.
4. Add the stock and bay leaf to the skillet and bring to a boil.
5. Reduce the heat to low, so the stock is simmering, and add the meatballs and cauliflower.
6. Simmer until the meatballs are cooked through and the cauliflower is tender-crisp, about 10 minutes.
7. Remove the bay leaf.
8. Top with cilantro and serve with flatbreads.

Serves 4. Prep time 15 minutes. Cook time 25 minutes.

Calories **259** / Calories from fat **95** / Total fat **10.6g** / Saturated fat **2.5g** / Trans fat **0.0g** / Sodium **900mg** / Carbs **23.9g** / Sugars **2.9g** / Protein **29.6g**

Crab and Celery Root Lettuce Cups

Gluten-free
Low-fat
Low-sodium
Nightshade-free

SNACKS

Crab is usually a very high-sodium ingredient so you might be surprised that this recipe is low-sodium. This is because of the relatively small amount of crab in each portion. Crab is often a very good choice for a healthy meal, despite the sodium, because it is also low in fat and calories. Crab is also a great source of protein and vitamin B_{12}.

Shopping tip Crab can be expensive, but you need only 4 ounces for these tasty appetizers. If you don't have a great source for fresh seafood, you can also get good quality canned crabmeat packed in water.

½ small celery root, washed, peeled, and grated

1 green onion, finely chopped

½ cup (about 4 ounces) cooked lump crabmeat, drained, shell pieces removed

2 tablespoons plain Greek yogurt

1 teaspoon fresh lime juice

1 teaspoon Dijon mustard

½ teaspoon finely chopped fresh thyme

Pinch of sea salt

Pinch of freshly ground black pepper

Pinch of cayenne pepper

12 small Boston lettuce leaves

1. In a medium bowl, stir together the celery root, green onion, and crabmeat.
2. In a small bowl, whisk together the yogurt, lime juice, mustard, thyme, salt, pepper, and cayenne until very well blended.
3. Add the yogurt mixture to the crab mixture and stir to mix.
4. Spoon about 3 teaspoons of filling into each lettuce leaf and serve immediately.

Makes 12 appetizers. Prep time 10 minutes.

Calories **16** / Calories from fat **2** / Total fat **0.4g** / Saturated fat **0.0g** / Trans fat **0.0g** / Sodium **53mg** / Carbs **2.0g** / Sugars **0.5g** / Protein **1.5g**

Maple Corn Muffins

These tender muffins might seem to have a lot of saturated fat in them, but it comes entirely from coconut oil, which is a healthy fat alternative. Saturated vegetable fats such as coconut oil do not have the same destructive effect as saturated animal fats. Coconut oil is burned very quickly in the body because it is composed mostly of medium-chain triglycerides rather than the long-chain fats found in butter and bacon fat. This means coconut oil is heart-friendly and is less likely to be stored as fat in the body.

Diet tip Substitute almond flour or spelt flour for the whole-wheat flour if you want a gluten-free recipe.

1½ cups cornmeal

1½ cups whole-wheat flour

1 tablespoon baking soda

1 teaspoon baking powder

Pinch of sea salt

2 eggs

½ cup pure maple syrup

½ cup almond milk

3 tablespoons coconut oil, melted

1 tablespoon apple cider vinegar

1 tablespoon pure vanilla extract

1. Preheat the oven to 350°F. Line a muffin tin with paper liners and set aside.
2. In a large bowl, combine the cornmeal, flour, baking soda, baking powder, and salt.
3. In a medium bowl, mix together the eggs, maple syrup, almond milk, coconut oil, vinegar, and vanilla until well blended.
4. Add the wet ingredients to the dry ingredients and stir until just combined.
5. Spoon the batter into the muffin cups until they are two-thirds full. Bake until a toothpick inserted in the center of a muffin comes out clean, about 15 minutes.
6. Cool the muffins completely before serving.

Makes 12 muffins. Prep time 5 minutes. Cook time 15 minutes.

Calories **214** / Calories from fat **66** / Total fat **7.3g** / Saturated fat **5.4g** / Trans fat **0.0g** / Sodium **355mg** / Carbs **33.4g** / Sugars **8.5g** / Protein **4.1g**

Spinach Dip

Gluten-free
Low-fat
Nightshade-free
Vegetarian

SNACKS

This version of spinach dip is much lower in fat and calories than the traditional sour cream and mayonnaise recipe. Make sure you don't skip blanching the spinach in this recipe, because cooking your spinach makes the nutrients more available for the body. This means cooked spinach is healthier than raw!

Shopping tip To save time, you can buy a good-quality frozen chopped spinach instead of blanching your own. Make sure you thaw it completely and squeeze out all the liquid before adding the spinach to the rest of the ingredients, or your dip will be watery.

2 cups packed spinach leaves

1 cup cottage cheese

1 green onion, cut into 1-inch pieces

1 tablespoon chopped fresh parsley

1 teaspoon minced garlic

Freshly ground black pepper

1. Fill a medium saucepan with water and bring the water to a boil over medium-high heat.
2. Add the spinach and blanch until tender, about 2 minutes.
3. Drain the spinach and run it under cold water.
4. Squeeze as much water as possible out of the blanched spinach.
5. In a food processor, combine the spinach, cottage cheese, green onion, parsley, and garlic and pulse until blended but not smooth.
6. Transfer the spinach mixture to a medium bowl and season with pepper to taste.
7. Cover the dip, and put it in the refrigerator until you are ready to serve it.
8. Serve with vegetables or baked pita bread.

Serves 6. Prep time 5 minutes. Cook time 25 minutes.

Calories **40** / Calories from fat **8** / Total fat **0.8g** / Saturated fat **0.0g** / Trans fat **0.0g** / Sodium **162mg** / Carbs **2.1g** / Sugar **0.0g** / Protein **5.6g**

Gluten-free
Low-fat
Low-sodium
Vegan
Vegetarian

SNACKS

Sweet Potato Hummus

This very tasty, slightly sweet hummus is an absolutely glorious reddish orange color. The texture is very close to the traditional chickpea version, so try it as a spread on wraps and sandwiches as well as a veggie and pita dip. You can even toss it with whole-grain pasta for a delicious, simple meal.

Diet tip If you need to follow a FODMAP-free diet, remove the maple syrup and enjoy this dip with vegetables on the approved list, like cucumbers, carrots, and green beans.

2 large sweet potatoes

1 large red bell pepper

Olive oil

¼ cup fresh lemon juice

1 teaspoon cumin

1 teaspoon pure maple syrup

½ teaspoon minced garlic

Pinch of cayenne pepper

Sea salt

1. Preheat the oven to 350°F. Line a baking tray with foil.
2. Prick the sweet potatoes with a fork and lightly coat the red pepper with olive oil.
3. Place the potatoes and pepper on the baking tray and bake until they are soft.
4. After about 20 minutes, remove the pepper from the oven and put it in a small bowl. Cover the bowl tightly with plastic wrap and set aside while the potatoes continue to bake, about another 20 minutes.
5. Remove the potatoes from the oven and let them cool for about 10 minutes. Then scoop out the flesh into a food processor.
6. Carefully remove the pepper from the bowl, peel off the skin, remove the seeds, and place the flesh in the food processor with the sweet potatoes.
7. Add the remaining ingredients and pulse until the hummus is smooth.
8. Transfer the mixture to a serving bowl and refrigerate for at least an hour until cool.
9. Serve with cut-up vegetables.

Serves 6. Prep time 5 minutes. Cook time 45 minutes.

Calories **75** / Calories from fat **3** / Total fat **0.3g** / Saturated fat **0.0g** / Trans fats **0.0g** / Sodium **8mg** / Carbs **16.8g** / Sugars **2.3g** / Protein **1.2g**

Fresh Fruit Salsa

This salsa is not too sweet, despite the fruit, and has a definite kick from the jalapeño pepper and green onion. Peaches are consistently on the "dirty dozen" list of pesticide-contaminated produce. Make sure you buy organic whenever possible and thoroughly scrub your peaches before using them.

Cooking tip Your peaches and mango should be just ripe or even a little green, so that this salsa is not mushy. If they are too ripe, use them for another dish or eat them cut up as a snack.

2 large ripe peaches, peeled, pitted, and cut into chunks
½ mango, peeled, pitted, and cut into chunks
1 large tomato, cut into 8 wedges
1 green onion, coarsely chopped

1 jalapeño pepper, chopped with the seeds
½ cup fresh cilantro
1 tablespoon minced garlic
1 teaspoon fresh lime juice
Baked tortilla chips or pita bread

1. In a food processor, combine the peaches, mango, tomatoes, onion, jalapeño, cilantro, garlic, and lime juice and pulse until the salsa is coarsely chopped but not completely smooth. Scrape down the sides of the bowl at least once.
2. Transfer to a serving bowl and serve with tortilla chips or pita bread.

Serves 6. Prep time 15 minutes.

Calories **44** / Calories from fat **2** / Total fat **0.3g** / Saturated fat **0.0g** / Trans fats **0.0g** / Sodium **3mg** / Carbs **9.9g** / Sugars **8.0g** / Protein **1.1g**

Southwestern Bean Dip

Bean dips are usually fatty and ooze with cheese, which does not fit into your eating clean diet. But this healthy recipe is just as tasty as its calorie-laden counterpart. There is no cheese in this dip; instead, there's a touch of tahini for a nutty, rich taste. Tahini is made from ground-up sesame seeds and is a great source of calcium, magnesium, and vitamins B_1, B_2, and E.

Shopping tip You will come across two kinds of tahini in your local grocery store: hulled and unhulled. Whenever possible, try to get unhulled tahini because leaving the hull on the sesame seeds when grinding them up makes the finished paste more nutritious.

2 cups canned sodium-free navy beans, rinsed and drained

1 cup homemade salsa

¼ cup tahini

Juice of 1 lime

1 teaspoon ground cumin

¼ teaspoon ground coriander

Pinch of crushed red pepper flakes

Baked tortilla chips or pita bread

1. In a food processor, combine the navy beans, salsa, tahini, lime juice, cumin, coriander, and pepper flakes and pulse until mixed but not completely smooth.
2. Scrape down the sides of the food processor and pulse until smooth.
3. Transfer to a serving bowl and serve with baked tortillas.

Serves 6. Prep time 5 minutes.

Calories **181** / Calories from fat **49** / Total fat **5.5g** / Saturated fat **0.8g** / Trans fat **0.0g** / Sodium **232mg** / Carbs **18.3g** / Sugars **2.7g** / Protein **12.4g**

Spinach and Sun-Dried Tomato–Stuffed Mushrooms

This is an elegant hors d'oeuvre that takes very little time to put together. Instead of button mushrooms, you can also use small portobellos or cremini mushrooms to change the taste and texture a little. Mushrooms are the only fruit or vegetable that are rich in vitamin D, so make sure you eat them regularly in the winter months, especially in the northern climates that have less daily sunshine exposure.

Cooking tip Oil-packed sun-dried tomatoes are delicious, but some people want to avoid the extra fat and calories. If you get the dried version without oil, soak them in water for at least an hour to plump them up.

16 large button mushrooms

1 tablespoon olive oil

1 green onion, finely chopped

1 tablespoon minced garlic

½ red bell pepper, seeded and finely chopped

¼ cup sun-dried tomatoes, finely diced

1 cup finely shredded baby spinach

½ cup finely chopped pecans

Freshly ground black pepper

1. Preheat the oven to 375°F. Line a baking sheet with foil.
2. Remove the stems from the mushrooms, creating a hollow, and set the stems aside. Place the mushrooms on the baking sheet, hollow side up.
3. Bake the mushroom caps for about 5 minutes until softened. Remove the caps from the oven and pour off any liquid that has purged from the mushrooms. Set aside.
4. Finely chop half the mushroom stems and set aside. Reserve the remaining half in a sealed bag to use in a stew or frittata.
5. In a skillet over medium-high heat, heat the oil and sauté the chopped mushroom caps, green onion, garlic, and red pepper until the vegetables are softened, about 3 minutes.

continued ➤

6. Add the sun-dried tomatoes and sauté for an additional minute.
7. Add the spinach and pecans to the skillet and stir until the spinach is wilted, about 3 minutes.
8. Remove the mixture from the heat and season with pepper to taste; stir to combine.
9. Spoon the filling into the mushroom caps and put them back in the oven for 5 minutes.
10. Serve warm, four per person.

Serves 4. Prep time 10 minutes. Cook time 20 minutes.

Calories **162** / Calories from fat **123** / Total fat **13.7g** / Saturated fat **1.3g** / Trans fat **0.0g** / Sodium **84mg** / Carbs **8.9g** / Sugars **4.2g** / Protein **5.2g**

Sesame-Crusted Chicken Tenders

You can eat these tempting golden strips as a filling snack with a dip, or as a light meal with a nice mixed green salad. They would be perfect after a workout because the chicken and sesame seeds are rich in the protein needed for muscle recovery. Protein is essential for building muscle tissue, and these tenders have over 40 grams per portion.

Leftovers tip If you have chicken tenders left over, simply store them in the refrigerator in a sealed plastic bag and use them in a pita or wrap the next day for lunch.

Nonstick olive oil cooking spray

1 egg white

1 tablespoon water

1 cup sesame seeds

12 chicken tenders, about 1 pound

1. Preheat the oven to 350°F. Line a baking sheet with foil and lightly coat it with the cooking spray; set aside.
2. In a small bowl, whisk the egg white and water together and set aside.
3. Put the sesame seeds on a small plate and set up next to the egg white mixture.
4. Pat the chicken dry with paper towels.
5. Dip a tender in the egg white mixture and allow the excess to drip off. Then dredge the chicken in the sesame seeds to coat completely.
6. Place the coated tender on the baking sheet.
7. Repeat with the remaining tenders.
8. Lightly spray the tenders with the cooking spray and bake until the chicken is cooked through and the tenders are light golden brown, turning once, about 15 minutes.
9. Serve three per person with a salad or your favorite clean eating dip.

Serves 4. Prep time 5 minutes. Cook time 15 minutes.

Calories **397** / Calories from fat **197** / Total fat **21.9g** / Saturated fat **2.5g** / Trans fat **0.0g** / Sodium **149mg** / Carbs **8.5g** / Sugar **0.0g** / Protein **43.7g**

Avocado Stuffed with Chicken Salad

The pastel green of the avocado, white chicken, and flecks of orange carrot and red pepper combine to create visual and culinary appeal. If your avocado halves do not have very deep cavities when you remove the pits, carefully scoop out a bit more flesh so there is room for the chicken salad. Use the scooped-out avocado in a smoothie or dip.

Cooking tip Chicken breast is a popular ingredient in clean eating. To save time, bake four or five breasts at the beginning of the week and store them in the refrigerator in a sealed container for when you need them.

1 cup finely chopped cooked
    chicken breast
½ cup shredded carrot
1 red bell pepper, seeded and chopped
2 green onions, finely chopped
2 tablespoons chopped fresh cilantro

1 tablespoon fresh lemon juice
2 tablespoons Greek yogurt
Freshly ground black pepper, to taste
2 avocados, sliced in half lengthwise
    and pitted

1. In a medium bowl, mix together the chicken, carrot, red pepper, green onion, cilantro, lemon juice, yogurt, and pepper until well combined.
2. Spoon the chicken mixture into each avocado half and serve one avocado half per person.

Serves 4. Prep time 10 minutes.

Calories **291** / Calories from fat **192** / Total fat **21.4g** / Saturated fat **4.4g** / Trans fat **0.0g** / Sodium **64mg** / Carbs **12.7g** / Sugars **3.0g** / Protein **15.2g**

Cucumber Feta Dip

Gluten-free
Low-fat
Nightshade-free
Vegetarian

SNACKS

The flavor of this dish is so delicious you might want to eat it as a dip, spread, salad dressing, and maybe even on its own with just a spoon! The cucumber adds nice texture and a refreshing taste, along with the lemon juice. Lemon juice is packed with antioxidants and vitamin C, so it can help detoxify the body, boost the immune system, and improve digestion.

Nutrition tip Greek yogurt seems to be a healthy eating trend that is here to stay. It has twice the protein and less lactose than regular yogurt, because the whey is strained out.

2 cups plain Greek yogurt

¼ large English cucumber, grated, liquid squeezed out

¼ cup feta cheese

1 teaspoon minced garlic

3 teaspoons fresh lemon juice

3 teaspoons chopped fresh oregano

Freshly ground black pepper, to taste

1. In a large bowl, mix together all the ingredients until very well combined.
2. Cover the bowl and put it in the refrigerator until you are ready to serve.
3. Serve with pita bread or fresh cut vegetables.

Serves 4. Prep time 10 minutes.

Calories **128** / Calories from fat **60** / Total fat **6.7g** / Saturated fat **4.5g** / Trans fat **0.0g** / Sodium **144mg** / Carbs **6.6g** / Sugars **5.0g** / Protein **11.6g**

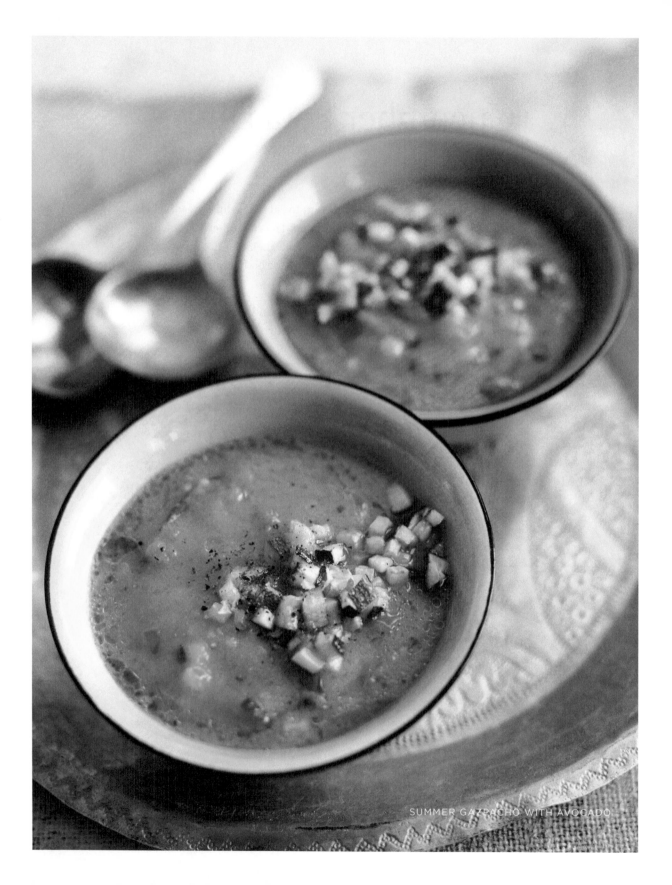

SUMMER GAZPACHO WITH AVOCADO

CHAPTER SEVEN

CHAPTER SEVEN

Soups and Salads

Gluten-free
Low-fat
Nightshade-free
Vegetarian

SOUPS AND
SALADS

Carrot Soup with Yogurt

Carrots are the superstars of this pretty soup, with very good reason. They are delicious, versatile, and packed with vitamins and other nutrients. Carrots contain a great deal of vitamin A (more than 200 percent of the daily recommended requirement), as well as vitamin C, iron, and calcium. Carrots promote healthy vision and can help prevent cancer.

1 teaspoon olive oil

½ small sweet onion, peeled and chopped

1½ pounds carrots, peeled and cut into
    1-inch chunks

3 cups fat-free, low-sodium
    vegetable stock

1 teaspoon grated fresh ginger

½ teaspoon ground nutmeg

Freshly ground black pepper

½ cup plain Greek yogurt

1. In a large saucepan over medium heat, heat the oil and sauté the onion until tender, about 3 minutes.
2. Add the carrots and stock and bring the mixture to a boil.
3. Reduce the heat to low and simmer until the carrots are tender, about 20 minutes.
4. Add the ginger and nutmeg and simmer for an additional 2 minutes.
5. Remove the mixture from the heat and purée the soup with an immersion blender or in a food processor until very smooth.
6. Season with pepper.
7. Serve topped with yogurt.

Serves 4. Prep time 10 minutes. Cook time 30 minutes.

Calories **114** / Calories from fat **22** / Total fat **2.4g** / Saturated fat **1.0g** / Trans fat **0.0g** / Sodium **464mg** / Carbs **19.1g** / Sugars **10.0g** / Protein **4.8g**

Rustic Tomato Soup

Gluten-free
Low-fat
Vegan
Vegetarian

SOUPS AND
SALADS

Homemade tomato soup rarely resembles the thin, flavorless, processed version most people are familiar with from childhood. This soup is rich with chunks of tomato, celery, and carrot, as well as an abundance of fresh herbs. Commercially produced hothouse tomatoes are often pale and flavorless. The best tomatoes for this soup are organic locally grown tomatoes—or better yet, grow your own!

Nutrition tip Did you know that tomatoes are actually healthier for you when cooked? Your body can absorb more of the lycopene in tomatoes after they are cooked.

1 teaspoon olive oil

1 sweet onion, peeled and diced

3 teaspoons minced garlic

2 celery stalks, diced

10 large ripe tomatoes, chopped

3 medium carrots, peeled and diced

4 cups fat-free, low-sodium
   vegetable stock

2 tablespoons chopped fresh basil

2 tablespoons chopped fresh parsley

1 teaspoon chopped fresh oregano

Freshly ground black pepper

1. In a large pot on medium heat, heat the olive oil and sauté the onion, garlic, and celery until softened, about 5 minutes.
2. Add the tomatoes, carrots, and stock and bring to a boil.
3. Reduce the heat to low and simmer the soup until the carrots are tender, about 25 minutes.
4. Remove the soup from the heat and purée with an immersion blender or in a food processor until the soup reaches the desired consistency. It is better a little chunky.
5. Stir in the basil, parsley, and oregano; season with pepper and serve warm.

Serves 4. Prep time 10 minutes. Cook time 30 minutes.

Calories **134** / Calories from fat **21** / Total fat **2.4g** / Saturated fat **0.0g** / Trans fat **0.0g** /
Sodium **112mg** / Carbs **30.0g** / Sugars **16.1g** / Protein **5.4g**

Gluten-free
Nightshade-free
Vegan
Vegetarian

SOUPS AND
SALADS

Roasted Beet Soup

Beets are an underused vegetable, mostly because many people have no idea what to do with them and beets can be very messy to prepare. Beets are a smart clean eating choice because they contain no saturated fat and no trans fat. They are also high in iron, fiber, and vitamins A and C. Beets can help fight cancer and protect you from heart disease.

Shopping tip Beets are available all year round in most areas, so try this soup in every season. When buying beets, try to get ones with the greens still attached so you can use the greens for a healthy, delicious salad. Detach the greens immediately and try to use them as soon as possible. The roots will keep for weeks in your refrigerator.

8 medium beets

½ small sweet onion, peeled and cut
    into chunks

2 garlic cloves, peeled

1 tablespoon olive oil

2 tablespoons apple cider vinegar

2 cups almond milk

¼ cup chopped fresh parsley

1. Preheat the oven to 350°F. Line a baking sheet with foil.
2. Peel the beets and cut them into quarters.
3. On the baking sheet, arrange the beets, onion, and garlic and drizzle the vegetables with the oil.
4. Bake until the beets are fork tender, about 35 minutes.
5. In a food processor, combine the vegetables, including any juices on the baking sheet, with the vinegar and almond milk, and process into a very smooth soup.
6. Serve warm, topped with parsley.

Serves 4. Prep time 10 minutes. Cook time 35 minutes.

Calories **152** / Calories from fat **55** / Total fat **6.1g** / Saturated fat **2.6g** / Trans fat **0.0g** / Sodium **159mg** / Carbs **25.5g** / Sugars **16.4g** / Protein **3.6g**

Cream of Vegetable Soup

Gluten-free
Nightshade-free
Vegan
Vegetarian

SOUPS AND
SALADS

Don't let the ingredient list of this recipe limit the vegetables you want to use. Pretty much any combination would taste fabulous, so try about seven or eight cups of chopped vegetables of any type. If you add potatoes, eggplant, or peppers to the mix, you can no longer consider the finished dish nightshade-free.

Nutrition tip Tofu is a great, inexpensive food that can make your sauces, soups, and smoothies lovely and creamy. It is high in protein, low in saturated fat, and low in calories.

1 teaspoon olive oil

¼ cup chopped sweet onion

2 celery stalks, diced

1 teaspoon minced garlic

4 cups fat-free, low-sodium
   vegetable stock

2 cups chopped cauliflower florets

1 cup chopped broccoli florets

1 cup shredded spinach

8 ounces silken tofu

1 teaspoon white wine vinegar

½ teaspoon ground nutmeg

Freshly ground black pepper

1. In a large pot over medium heat, heat the oil and sauté the onion, celery, and garlic until softened, about 3 minutes. Add the stock and bring the liquid to a boil.
2. Add the cauliflower and broccoli and reduce the heat to low so the soup simmers.
3. Cover the pot and cook until the vegetables are tender, about 25 minutes.
4. Add the spinach and simmer an additional 3 minutes.
5. Transfer the soup to a food processor and purée until it is smooth.
6. Add the tofu and vinegar and purée until the soup is very silky and smooth.
7. Season with the nutmeg and pepper to taste.
8. Serve warm.

Serves 6. Prep time 15 minutes. Cook time 40 minutes.

Calories **89** / Calories from fat **27** / Total fat **3.0g** / Saturated fat **0.0g** / Trans fat **0.0g** /
Sodium **126mg** / Carbs **8.1g** / Sugars **2.9g** / Protein **7.9g**

Summer Gazpacho with Avocado

Cold soups can be an acquired taste for those who have never tried them, but the fresh, unadulterated taste of vegetables and fruits can be addictive. The flavor of this soup is sharpened and brightened by a splash of fresh lemon juice and chopped cilantro. Try to use fresh vegetable juice whenever possible, and good, organic canned products if not, for the best taste.

Cooking tip Gazpacho is usually a chunky soup because the texture is part of the whole cold soup experience. If you enjoy a smoother soup, simply purée all the ingredients until you get the desired texture.

8 ripe plum tomatoes, chopped

1 large English cucumber, chopped

1 large red bell pepper, seeded
    and chopped

¼ small red onion, peeled and chopped

4 tablespoons chopped fresh cilantro

3 teaspoons fresh lemon juice

1 teaspoon minced garlic

Freshly ground black pepper, to taste

Hot pepper sauce

1 cup low-sodium prepared vegetable juice
    or fresh vegetable juice

1 ripe avocado, peeled and diced

1. In a food processor, combine all the ingredients except the juice and the avocado and process until well combined but still chunky.
2. Add the vegetable juice and pulse to combine to until the desired consistency is reached.
3. Store the soup in a sealed container in the refrigerator until you want to serve it.
4. Serve topped with chopped avocado.

Serves 4. Prep time 10 minutes. Cook time 30 minutes.

Calories **166** / Calories from fat **67** / Total fat **7.5g** / Saturated fat **1.0g** / Trans fat **0.0g** / Sodium **231mg** / Carbs **24.8g** / Sugars **13.7g** / Protein **5.0g**

Mango and Bean Salad

There is something decadent about ripe, luscious mango. Its texture is so silky and the flavor explodes in your mouth. Mango is high in fiber and vitamins A and C, and is also an excellent source of potassium and copper. This sunny fruit helps fight cancer, promotes great vision, and is excellent for the skin.

Shopping tip Prepared canned beans are usually a staple on clean eating diets because they are convenient, and there are many great organic sodium-free products available. You can certainly soak and cook your own, but the canned options will save time.

2 ripe mangoes, peeled, pitted, and diced

2 cups low-sodium black beans, rinsed
    well and drained

2 green onions, chopped finely

1 small red bell pepper, seeded and diced

1 large ripe tomato, seeded and diced

½ cup cooked barley

¼ cup chopped fresh cilantro

2 tablespoons fresh lime juice

Freshly ground black pepper, to taste

1. In a large bowl, combine all the ingredients.
2. Toss to mix and place in the refrigerator to chill for about 1 hour before serving.

Serves 6. Prep time 15 minutes.

Calories **239** / Calories from fat **49** / Total fat **5.4g** / Saturated fat **0.7g** / Trans fat **0.0g** / Sodium **207mg** / Carbs **38.0g** / Sugars **12.8g** / Protein **8.0g**

Low-sodium
Nightshade-free
Vegan
Vegetarian

SOUPS AND
SALADS

Moroccan Bulgur Salad

Texture and intense flavors are the hallmarks of this colorful, chunky main-dish salad that makes a filling, healthy lunch or snack. Bulgur is a wheat kernel that has been partially cooked and cracked. It is high in protein and fiber, low in sodium, and cholesterol-free.

Nutrition tip Bulgur is a fabulous substitute when you are tired of eating bowl after bowl of brown rice. It has twice the fiber and half the fat and calories of brown rice.

For the dressing:

3 tablespoons fresh lime juice

1 tablespoon olive oil

½ teaspoon ground cumin

¼ teaspoon ground coriander

¼ teaspoon ground cinnamon

Pinch of freshly ground black pepper

For the salad:

2 cups water

1½ cups uncooked bulgur, rinsed

2 cups canned low-sodium chickpeas, rinsed and drained

2 large carrots, peeled and shredded

½ cup dried cranberries

¼ cup slivered almonds

1 tablespoon chopped fresh mint

To make the dressing:

In a small bowl, whisk together all the dressing ingredients and set aside.

To make the salad:

1. In a medium saucepan over medium heat, combine the water and bulgur and bring to a boil.
2. Remove from the heat and cover the pot.
3. Let the bulgur sit for about 30 minutes until all the water is absorbed.
4. In a large bowl, combine the bulgur with the chickpeas, carrots, cranberries, almonds, and mint and toss.
5. Add the dressing and toss again until well mixed.
6. Cover the bowl and chill until you are ready to serve.

Serves 6. Prep time 15 minutes. Cook time 10 minutes.

Calories **239** / Calories from fat **49** / Total fat **5.4g** / Saturated fat **0.7g** / Trans fat **0.0g** / Sodium **40mg** / Carbs **56.3g** / Sugars **12.8g** / Protein **8.0g**

Shaved Asparagus Salad

There's a little extra prep here, but the effect is worth all the vegetable shaving involved in producing this salad. You want to try to get asparagus that is crisp and just thicker than a pencil. The thick asparagus might look easier to peel, but it can also be tough and bitter.

Cooking tip You can also grate your asparagus (on the coarsest grating surface) if you don't want to peel it. The salad will not have the same volume or elegant appearance as the shaved version, though.

3 bunches fresh asparagus,
   about 30 spears
1 tablespoon olive oil
1 small red onion, peeled and thinly sliced
2 tablespoons fresh orange juice

2 tablespoons fresh lemon juice
½ cup chopped pecans
½ cup shaved Parmesan cheese
2 tablespoons chopped fresh thyme
Freshly ground black pepper

1. Trim the woody ends off the asparagus.
2. Lay an asparagus stalk on a cutting board and shave off long ribbons with a vegetable peeler until the stalk is used up. Repeat with all the spears.
3. In a large bowl, toss the asparagus ribbons with the olive oil.
4. Add the onion, orange juice, and lemon juice and toss to combine.
5. Add the pecans, Parmesan cheese, and thyme.
6. Season with pepper.
7. Serve immediately or store the salad in an airtight container in the refrigerator for up to 6 hours.

Serves 6. Prep time 30 minutes.

Calories **145** / Calories from fat **98** / Total fat **10.9g** / Saturated fat **2.2g** / Trans fat **0.0g** /
Sodium **117mg** / Carbs **7.7g** / Sugars **3.7g** / Protein **6.2g**

Cobb Salad

This main meal salad is high in protein but not too filling, so it is ideal before playing sports or engaging in an activity-packed afternoon. This recipe omits the bacon, cheese, and creamy dressing often found in the original Cobb salad, but none of the taste. Try different greens, such as spinach and peppery arugula, to create delicious variations.

Cooking tip You will find many uses for hardboiled eggs when eating clean. In the interest of saving time, boil a dozen at the beginning of the week and store them in the shells, in the egg carton, in your refrigerator until you need them.

For the dressing:

¼ cup balsamic vinegar

1 teaspoon honey

¼ cup olive oil

Freshly ground black pepper, to taste

For the salad:

6 cups chopped romaine hearts

2 large ripe tomatoes, chopped

2 large hardboiled eggs, peeled and sliced

One 6-ounce cooked boneless, skinless chicken breast, chopped

1 ripe avocado, peeled, pitted, and cut into ½ inch slices

To make the dressing:

In a small bowl, whisk together all the dressing ingredients and set aside.

To make the salad:

1. In a large bowl, combine all the salad ingredients and toss.
2. Arrange the salad on plates and drizzle with dressing.
3. Serve immediately.

Serves 6. Prep time 15 minutes.

Calories **243** / Calories from fat **163** / Total fat **18.1g** / Saturated fat **3.1g** / Trans fat **0.0g** / Sodium **72mg** / Carbs **8.3g** / Sugars **2.9g** / Protein **15.4g**

Asian Slaw

Gluten-free
Low-fat
Nightshade-free
Vegan
Vegetarian

SOUPS AND
SALADS

Jicama is an important ingredient in this salad because it has the most interesting crisp, juicy texture and a slightly sweet taste. It is a member of the potato family and can be eaten raw or cooked. Jicama is high in vitamin C, fiber, iron, potassium, and calcium, and extremely low in fat and sodium.

Shopping tip When purchasing jicama, look for medium-size vegetables, about three to four inches across, with no wet or soft spots. Never buy jicama that has been refrigerated or store them in the refrigerator, because temperatures lower than 50°F can reduce their shelf life.

1 small head red cabbage, shredded

2 medium carrots, peeled and shredded

1 jicama, peeled and shredded

2 apples, cored and diced

2 tablespoons fresh lemon juice

1 tablespoon sesame oil

1 tablespoon grated ginger

1 teaspoon minced garlic

½ cup toasted unsalted cashews

1. In a large bowl, combine the cabbage, carrots, jicama, and apples and toss until well mixed.
2. In a small bowl, whisk together the lemon juice, sesame oil, ginger, and garlic.
3. Add the dressing and cashews to the vegetables and toss again.
4. Put the slaw in the refrigerator for at least 1 hour before serving to let the flavors blend.

Serves 4. Prep time 20 minutes.

Calories **302** / Calories from fat **107** / Total fat **11.9g** / Saturated fat **2.2g** / Trans fat **0.0g** / Cholesterol **0mg** / Sodium **72mg** / Carbs **47.4g** / Sugars **20.4g** / Protein **6.3g**

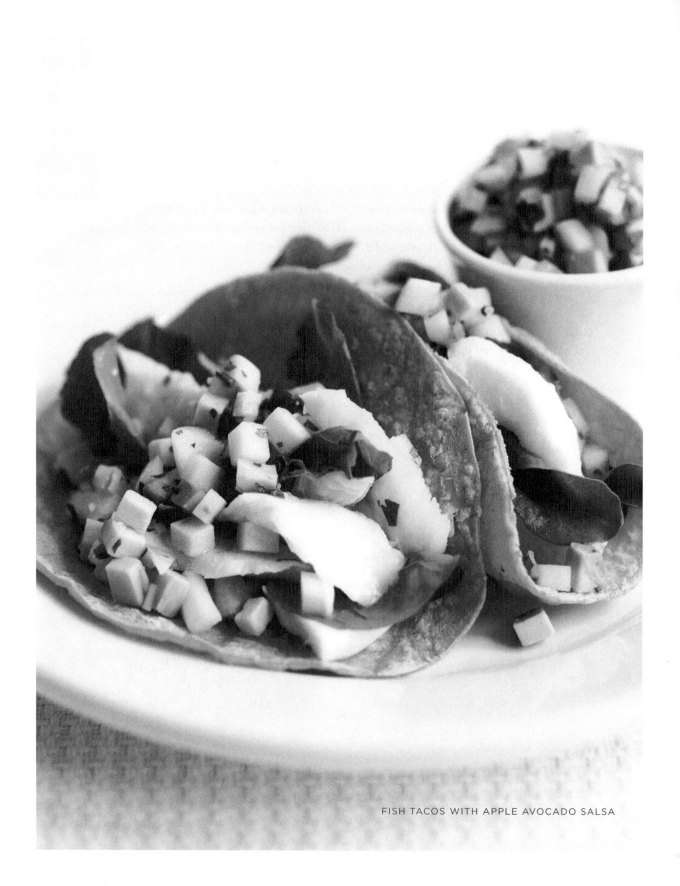

FISH TACOS WITH APPLE AVOCADO SALSA

CHAPTER EIGHT

Sandwiches and Wraps

Tabbouleh Pita

Tabbouleh is usually served as a salad, but it is a great sandwich stuffer. A main flavor component in this dish is parsley, and this herb also provides health benefits. Parsley is very high in vitamin K and flavonoids, especially luteolin, which helps fight free radicals in the body. This popular herb can help protect against heart disease, rheumatoid arthritis, and stroke.

Cooking tip Always chop parsley with a very sharp knife so you don't crush and bruise the tender leaves. Damaged parsley will smell like moldy grass in as little as a day, and will not taste nice, either.

4 whole-wheat pitas

1 cup uncooked bulgur, rinsed and drained

2 cups hot water

3 tablespoons olive oil

Juice of 1 lemon

1 teaspoon minced garlic

3 green onions, finely chopped

2 large tomatoes, diced

1 medium English cucumber, finely diced

1 large red bell pepper, seeded and diced

½ cup finely chopped fresh parsley

1. Cut the pitas in half and pry them open. Set aside.
2. Into a large bowl, add the bulgur first and then the hot water.
3. Soak for 15 minutes and then drain the remaining water out of the bowl.
4. Add the remaining ingredients to the bulgur and stir to thoroughly combine.
5. Divide the bulgur salad evenly among the pita halves and serve.

Serves 4. Prep time 15 minutes.

Calories **428** / Calories from fat **118** / Total fat **13.1g** / Saturated fat **1.9g** / Trans fat **0.0g** / Sodium **364mg** / Carbs **56.0g** / Sugars **5.1g** / Protein **12.7g**

Fish Tacos with Apple Avocado Salsa

Gluten-free
Low-fat
Low-sodium
Nightshade-free

SANDWICHES
AND WRAPS

Traditional tacos are actually made with soft corn tortillas. If you prefer to buy hard taco shells, make sure you get ones that are low in sodium. Corn tortillas are high in fiber, phosphorus, copper, and manganese. They can also be a bit high in calories, and you won't want to use them for every sandwich and wrap.

Leftovers tip You will only be using half an avocado in this recipe, so it is important to preserve the other half for another recipe. Leave the skin on and the pit in the side of the fruit that you are storing. Place the avocado in an airtight container with a quarter of a peeled onion. The sulfur from the onion will keep the cut edges of the avocado from browning for up to three days in the fridge.

For the salsa:

1 small Macintosh apple, peeled, cored,
    and diced
½ avocado, peeled, pitted, and diced
¼ small sweet onion, diced
1 tablespoon chopped fresh cilantro
1 tablespoon freshly squeezed lime juice
Sea salt
Freshly ground black pepper

For the tacos:

2 tablespoons balsamic vinegar
2 tablespoons chopped fresh cilantro
Juice of ½ lime
1 teaspoon olive oil
1 teaspoon honey
6 ounces halibut fillets
Four 6-inch corn tortillas
¼ cup baby spinach

To make the salsa:

1. In a small bowl, stir together the apple, avocado, onion, cilantro, and lime juice.
2. Season with salt and pepper.
3. Set the salsa aside, covered in the fridge, until you need it.

continued ➤

To make the tacos:

1. In a small bowl, whisk together the balsamic vinegar, cilantro, lime juice, olive oil, and honey.
2. Add the fish to the balsamic mixture and marinate for 15 minutes.
3. In a small skillet over medium-high heat, cook the marinated fish (but not the extra marinade remaining in the bowl), turning once, until it flakes when cut with a fork, about 3 minutes per side.
4. Place the tortillas on a clean work surface and divide the salsa evenly between them.
5. Add the spinach to each tortilla.
6. Divide the fish evenly between the tortillas.
7. Fold the tortillas over the fish and serve warm.
8. Place the tortillas on a clean work surface and divide the slaw evenly between them. Divide the fish evenly between the tortillas.
9. Fold the tortillas over the fish and serve warm.

Serves 2. Prep time 15 minutes. Cook time 6 minutes.

Calories **409** / Calories from fat **144** / Total fat **16.0g** / Saturated fat **3.0g** / Trans fat **0.0g** / Sodium **206mg** / Carbs **41.9g** / Sugars **12.1g** / Protein **26.7g**

Baked Pita Pockets
with Tuna and Avocado

This is an extremely simple dish with few ingredients that can be thrown together in less than fifteen minutes. You don't have to bake this wrap if you are in a rush—simply stuff and run! Avocado provides a lovely creaminess to the tuna that is usually achieved in sandwiches with gobs of mayonnaise. You will love this healthier version of an old favorite.

Shopping tip Avocado is a fruit that does not ripen while on the tree. It ripens after it is picked, so you might buy an unripe one. When you get home, put it in a paper bag with an apple or a banana. These fruits naturally produce a fruit gas called ethylene, which will speed up the ripening process.

Four 6-inch whole-wheat pitas, halved and pried opened

1½ cups canned water-packed tuna, drained

1 large tomato, thinly sliced

½ avocado, peeled, pitted, and diced

4 ounces alfalfa sprouts

1. Preheat the oven to 350°F.
2. Place the pita bread on a clean work surface and spoon the tuna, divided evenly, into each of the halves.
3. Top each mound of tuna with a quarter of the tomato and avocado.
4. Place the pita halves on a baking sheet and bake about 5 minutes, or until lightly browned.
5. Add the sprouts and serve immediately.

Serves 4. Prep time 10 minutes. Cook time 5 minutes.

Calories **283** / Calories from fat **59** / Total fat **6.6g** / Saturated fat **1.1g** / Trans fat **0.0g** / Sodium **394mg** / Carbs **19.9g** / Sugars **2.4g** / Protein **30.3g**

Spinach and Bean Burrito Wraps

Beans and rice are a traditional food combination in many cultures around the world, because they are nutritious and relatively inexpensive. They are both high in iron and vitamin B, and when served together they create a complete protein with all nine essential amino acids. You can use other beans in this wrap, such as red beans and even lentils, if that is what is in your pantry.

Diet tip If you serve this wrap without the yogurt or substitute with an almond product, it can be a great vegan lunch or snack.

Four 8-inch whole-grain tortillas

4 cups shredded baby spinach

2 cups cooked black beans, rinsed and drained

1 cup cooked brown rice

½ cup chopped romaine lettuce

½ cup homemade salsa

¼ cup plain Greek yogurt

1. Preheat the oven to 250°F.
2. Place the tortillas in a stack and wrap them in in foil. Put them into the oven to warm.
3. In a large skillet over medium heat, heat the spinach and black beans, stirring, until the spinach and beans are warmed through, about 4 minutes.
4. Take the warm tortillas out of the oven and spread them out on a clean work space. Spoon the spinach mixture, divided evenly, in the center of each tortilla.
5. Spread the rice, lettuce, salsa, and yogurt, divided evenly, over the spinach mixture.
6. Roll up the wraps and serve warm.

Serves 4. Prep time 15 minutes. Cook time 5 minutes.

Calories **490** / Calories from fat **61** / Total fat **7.5g** / Saturated fat **2.1g** / Trans fat **0.0g** / Sodium **551mg** / Carbs **83.1g** / Sugars **4.0g** / Protein **25.2g**

Turkey and Sun-Dried Tomato Wraps

Turkey is sometimes passed over in favor of chicken because many people associate this bird with huge, gut-busting dinners and days spent in the gym to overcome overeating. Turkey breast is considerably lower in calories and fat than chicken breast and contains no saturated fat. The downside of turkey can be that it is also higher in sodium and lower in protein than chicken, but turkey is still a healthy clean eating option.

Cooking tip You can use up leftover turkey breast in this wrap after Thanksgiving and Christmas dinner.

1 large ripe tomato, chopped

1 cup fresh or frozen (and thawed)
    corn kernels

¼ cup chopped sun-dried tomatoes

Four 6-inch multigrain tortillas

Eight ¼-inch slices low-sodium deli
    turkey breast

2 cups shredded spinach

1. In a large bowl, stir together the tomato, corn, and sun-dried tomatoes until well mixed.
2. Place the tortillas on a clean work surface and top each one with two slices of turkey. Spoon the corn mixture, divided evenly, onto the turkey and top each tortilla with with ½ cup of spinach.
3. Roll up the wraps and serve.

Serves 4. Prep time 15 minutes.

Calories **203** / Calories from fat **30** / Total fat **3.4g** / Saturated fat **0.9g** / Trans fat **0.0g** / Sodium **543mg** / Carbs **36.2g** / Sugars **6.7g** / Protein **15.6g**

Chicken Caprese Wraps

Insalata Caprese is a simple salad of basil, fresh mozzarella cheese, and tomato served as an antipasto in Italy and other countries. This wrap takes those perfectly balanced components and adds chicken and a splash of balsamic vinegar to intensify the flavors. You can omit the chicken for a vegetarian meal and still have a filling and nutritious lunch.

Shopping tip Try fresh mozzarella cheese with this dish, if you can find a good source that uses whole milk. Keep in mind that fresh mozzarella should be eaten within a day of purchasing it because it is very perishable.

1 tablespoon balsamic vinegar

1 teaspoon minced garlic

Pinch of freshly ground black pepper

4 cups chopped romaine lettuce

2 cups cherry tomatoes, halved

Two 5-ounce cooked, skinless, boneless chicken breasts, shredded

2 tablespoons chopped or shredded fresh mozzarella cheese

½ cup chopped fresh basil

Four 6-inch gluten-free whole-wheat tortillas

1. In a large bowl, whisk together the balsamic vinegar, garlic, and pepper.
2. Add the lettuce, cherry tomatoes, chicken, cheese, and basil to the bowl and toss to combine.
3. Place the tortillas on a clean work space, and scoop about 1 cup of the chicken mixture onto each tortilla.
4. Roll up the tortillas and serve.

Serves 4. Prep time 15 minutes.

Calories **233** / Calories from fat **40** / Total fat **4.5g** / Saturated fat **1.4g** / Trans fat **0.0g** / Sodium **184mg** / Carbs **31.0g** / Sugars **3.1g** / Protein **22.1g**

Grilled Vegetable Buns

Low-fat
Low-sodium
Vegan
Vegetarian

SANDWICHES
AND WRAPS

This crusty, lightly toasted Italian bun is heaped with warm, slightly sweet grilled vegetables, along with ripe, juicy tomatoes and a splash of tart balsamic vinegar. The juices soak into the soft parts of the bread, and every bite is an explosion of flavor.

Cooking tip If you are in the mood for a salad instead of a sandwich, use this recipe for two portions and omit the bun. Or you can just use the bun to soak up all the juices on your plate.

1 small eggplant, cut into 8 slices about ¼-inch thick

2 red bell peppers, halved and seeded

1 small red onion, peeled and cut into ¼-inch-thick slices

1 green zucchini, cut lengthwise into 4 long pieces

Freshly ground black pepper, to taste

2 tablespoons olive oil, divided

2 tablespoons balsamic vinegar

4 ciabatta buns, split

2 ripe tomatoes, cut into 8 slices about ¼ inch thick

1. Preheat a barbecue grill to medium-high, or preheat the broiler.
2. In a large bowl, combine the eggplant, red pepper, red onion, zucchini, and black pepper with 1 tablespoon of the oil, and toss gently until well coated.
3. On the barbecue, grill the vegetables until tender and lightly charred on each side, about 6 minutes. Or in the oven, place the vegetables in a flat pan under the broiler, turning once, until tender and lightly charred, about 6 minutes.
4. In a large bowl, toss the grilled vegetables with the balsamic vinegar, and set aside.
5. Brush the bun halves with the remaining tablespoon of oil and place each half cut-side down on the grill, or cut-side up in the broiler.
6. Grill or broil for 1 minute and remove from the heat.
7. Top the bun bottoms with tomato slices and an assortment of the grilled vegetables, and top with the other half of the bun.
8. Serve warm.

Serves 4. Prep time 15 minutes. Cook time 7 minutes.

Calories **234** / Calories from fat **84** / Total fat **9.4g** / Saturated fat **1.0g** / Trans fat **0.0g** / Sodium **14mg** / Carbs **31.4g** / Sugars **9.3g** / Protein **7.4g**

FODMAP-free
Low-fat
Vegan
Vegetarian

SANDWICHES
AND WRAPS

Vegetarian Hummus Club Sandwiches

The club sandwich is more than one hundred years old and can be found in a dizzying range of dining establishments, from diners to four-star restaurants. There are many variations on the traditional chicken, bacon, tomato, and lettuce, including this tasty hummus club recipe. All real clubs have three pieces of bread stacked perfectly with other ingredient layers, all held together by toothpicks.

Shopping tip Look for reduced-calorie bread that is thinner and has air added during the production process, which produces slices that are about 50 calories each instead of 110 in standard bread slices.

Twelve 1-ounce slices whole-wheat or
  multigrain bread
1 cup homemade hummus
2 cups shredded Boston lettuce

2 large ripe tomatoes, sliced into 8 slices,
  about ¼-inch thick
1 small red onion, peeled and thinly sliced
1 large English cucumber, thinly sliced

1. Place 4 slices of bread on a clean work surface.
2. Spread 2 tablespoons of hummus evenly on each piece of bread.
3. Top the hummus with ¼ cup lettuce, 2 tomato slices, a couple of onion slices, and some sliced cucumber.
4. Place another piece of bread on top of the cucumber and spread 2 tablespoons of hummus on each piece of bread.
5. Top the second piece of bread with ¼ cup lettuce, 2 tomato slices, and a couple of onion and cucumber slices.
6. Top with the last pieces of bread and secure the sandwiches with toothpicks.
7. Cut each sandwich into four pieces diagonally, so that a toothpick is in each of the pieces, and serve.

Serves 4. Prep time 20 minutes.

Calories **262** / Calories from fat **35** / Total fat **3.9g** / Saturated fat **0.8g** / Trans fat **0.0g** / Sodium **361mg** / Carbs **58.0g** / Sugars **9.0g** / Protein **12.8g**

Tropical Chicken-Salad Wraps

The tart sweetness of the pineapple is lovely with chicken for a refreshing lunch or light dinner. Pineapple is not a single fruit but rather a bunch of small fruits around a core. You can see each fruit in the "eyes" that create the rough, scaly surface of the pineapple.

Cooking tip Make sure you squeeze out the pineapple very well or the wraps will be soggy. Reserve the pineapple juice for a smoothie, dressings, or marinades.

1 cup chopped, cooked chicken breast

½ cup crushed unsweetened canned pineapple, drained

3 tablespoons almond slivers

3 tablespoons Greek yogurt

1 tablespoon chopped green onion

Freshly ground black pepper

Two 8-inch whole-grain tortillas

½ cup shredded lettuce

1. In a medium bowl, mix the chicken, pineapple, almonds, yogurt, and green onion together.
2. Season the mixture with pepper.
3. Place the tortillas on a clean work surface and spoon the chicken filling into the center of each tortilla.
4. Top each tortilla with ¼ cup of shredded lettuce and roll the tortilla up.
5. Serve 1 tortilla per person.

Serves 2. Prep time 15 minutes.

Calories **320** / Calories from fat **87** / Total fat **9.7g** / Saturated fat **1.6g** / Trans fat **0.0g** / Sodium **275mg** / Carbs **26.1g** / Sugars **11.7g** / Protein **33.2g**

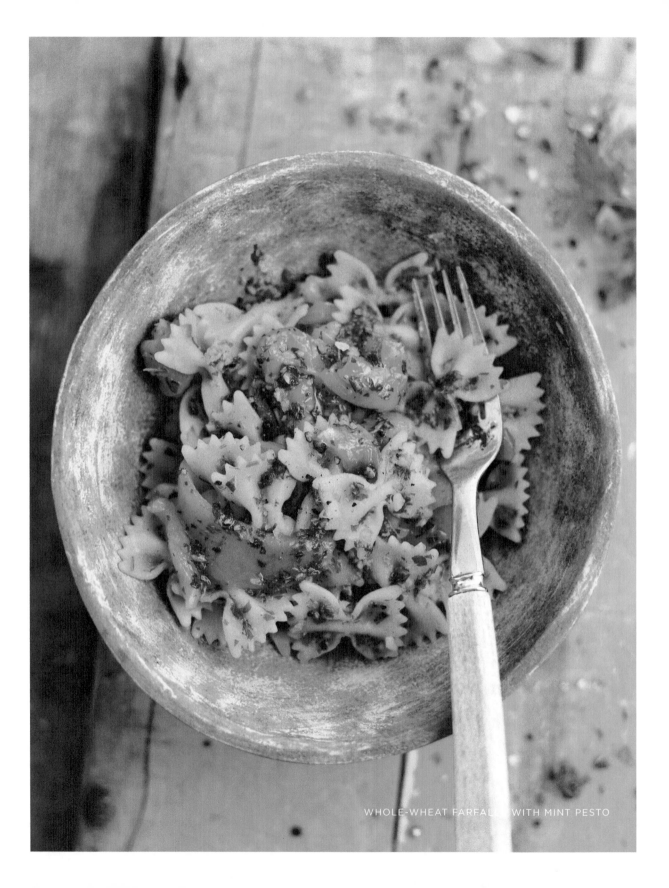

WHOLE-WHEAT FARFALLE WITH MINT PESTO

CHAPTER NINE

Side Dishes

Grilled Corn with Garlic

If you have never tried cooking corn on the barbeque, this recipe will be a revelation. Corn gets plump, juicy, and deliciously caramelized over open flames. If you don't have a grill, you can make corn in your broiler and it will still taste great. Corn has about 80 calories an ear, and is high in fiber and low in fat. Corn helps stabilize blood sugar, promotes healthy vision, and can help prevent heart disease.

Shopping tip If you shuck your corn before buying it in the supermarket, make sure you transfer it to a resealable plastic bag when you get home, to keep it fresh. You can keep corn in the refrigerator for up to five days if it is stored correctly.

4 teaspoons butter

2 teaspoons minced garlic

4 ears fresh corn on the cob, shucked

2 tablespoons grated Parmesan cheese

4 teaspoons chopped fresh parsley

Freshly ground black pepper

1. Preheat the barbecue to medium-high heat or preheat the broiler.
2. In a small saucepan over medium heat, melt the butter and sauté the garlic until soft, about 3 minutes.
3. Remove the pan from the heat and brush the garlic butter onto the corn.
4. On the barbecue, grill the corn, turning to grill all sides, until slightly charred and tender crisp, 10 to 20 minutes. Or in the oven, put the corn under the broiler for 15 to 20 minutes, turning about every 5 minutes.
5. Serve the corn topped with the cheese, parsley, and sprinkling of pepper.

Serves 4. Prep time 5 minutes. Cook time 15 minutes.

Calories **140** / Calories from fat **66** / Total fat **7.3g** / Saturated fat **4.5g** / Trans fat **0.0g** / Sodium **159mg** / Carbs **15.2g** / Sugars **2.3g** / Protein **6.6g**

Pico de Gallo Black Beans

This is a perfect side dish for a spicy grilled chicken or pork entrée. It can even be a main course if you are looking for a meat-free dish. The lovely citrusy and slightly nutty flavor of this dish comes from the cumin. Cumin is not just a fabulous seasoning; it is also a great source of iron, calcium, magnesium, and manganese. This means it can boost the immune system and promote healthy digestion.

Diet tip If you are following a vegan diet, leave out the feta cheese topping; this dish is already packed with protein.

1 cup dried black beans, rinsed and
    picked through

½ small sweet onion, finely chopped

1 teaspoon minced garlic

1 teaspoon ground cumin

1 teaspoon ground coriander

1 small ripe tomato, chopped

4 teaspoons finely chopped red bell pepper

4 teaspoons finely chopped red onion

¼ cup low-sodium feta cheese

1. In a medium bowl, cover the beans with water to about 1 inch above the level of the beans and soak in the refrigerator overnight. Drain the beans before using.
2. In a medium saucepan over medium-high heat, combine the beans with the onion, garlic, cumin, coriander, and 3 cups of water, and bring to a boil.
3. Reduce the heat to low and simmer until the beans are very tender, about 35 minutes.
4. While the beans are cooking, in a medium bowl make the pico de gallo by mixing together the tomato, red pepper, and red onion until well combined. Set aside.
5. Drain the beans and spoon them onto individual plates.
6. Serve topped with the pico de gallo and feta cheese.

Serves 4. Prep time 20 minutes, plus soaking time. Cook time 40 minutes.

Calories **186** / Calories from fat **17** / Total fat **1.9g** / Saturated fat **0.8g** / Trans fat **0.0g** / Sodium **110mg** / Carbs **33.1g** / Sugars **2.3g** / Protein **12.7g**

FODMAP-free
Gluten-free
Low-fat
Nightshade-free
Vegan
Vegetarian

SIDE DISHES

Roasted Vegetables with Thyme

The scent of gently caramelizing vegetables roasting in the oven will likely call your family to dinner long before you are ready to put it on the table. Try to cut the various root vegetables in similar sizes so they roast evenly, and make sure you toss them with the other ingredients thoroughly enough to coat every piece.

Shopping tip Don't be put off by the strange, dirty, bulbous appearance of the celery root (celeriac), because under the skin is a potato-like vegetable with a mild, pleasant celery taste. It is available year round, but is best in the late fall and winter months.

1 small butternut squash, peeled and cut into 1-inch cubes

2 carrots, peeled and cut into 1-inch chunks

3 parsnips, peeled and cut into 1-inch chunks

1 small celeriac root, peeled and cut into 1-inch chunks

1 large sweet potato, peeled and cut into 1-inch chunks

2 tablespoons olive oil

2 teaspoons chopped fresh thyme

Freshly ground black pepper, to taste

1. Preheat the oven to 400°F. Line a baking sheet with foil and set aside.
2. In a large bowl, toss together all the ingredients.
3. Transfer the vegetables to the prepared baking sheet and bake until they are tender and lightly browned, stirring occasionally, about 45 minutes.
4. Serve warm.

Serves 4. Prep time 10 minutes. Cook time 45 minutes.

Calories **231** / Calories from fat **68** / Total fat **7.5g** / Saturated fat **1.1g** / Trans fat **0.0g** / Sodium **75mg** / Carbs **42.3g** / Sugars **11.2g** / Protein **3.6g**

Spiced Squash Casserole

The prep is a bit more involved for this casserole than for many of the other recipes in this book—you double-process the squash—but the end result is smooth, luscious, and naturally sweet. Well worth the effort! Butternut squash is what's listed in the recipe, but any winter squash (except spaghetti) will do. Just make sure you have about eight cups of cubed squash.

Cooking tip Cutting winter squash in half can be a dangerous and difficult task, because it is so hard and the curved surface of the vegetable makes it likely to roll. Try placing the whole squash in the microwave about two minutes before cutting it, to make this process easier and safer.

Nonstick cooking spray

1 large butternut squash, cut in half and seeded

½ cup canned low-fat coconut milk

2 eggs

2 tablespoons pure maple syrup

4 teaspoons cornstarch

1 teaspoon ground cinnamon

¼ teaspoon ground nutmeg

¼ teaspoon ground cloves

1. Preheat the oven to 400°F. Line a baking sheet with foil and lightly coat the foil with cooking spray.
2. Place the squash cut-side down on the baking sheet and bake until the squash is tender and collapsed, about 30 minutes.
3. Remove the squash from the oven and let it cool for about 10 minutes.
4. Reduce the oven temperature to 350°F.
5. Scoop out the flesh of the squash with a spoon.
6. In a food processor, process the squash with the remaining ingredients until smooth, scraping down the sides of the bowl at least once.
7. Spoon the squash mixture into a casserole and bake until the mixture is set, about 35 minutes.
8. Serve warm.

Serves 8. Prep time 5 minutes. Cook time 1 hour and 10 minutes.

Calories **132** / Calories from fat **45** / Total fat **5.0g** / Saturated fat **3.6g** / Trans fat **0.0g** / Sodium **25mg** / Carbs **22.2g** / Sugars **8.8g** / Protein **3.0g**

Gluten-free
Low-sodium
Nightshade-free
Vegan
Vegetarian

SIDE DISHES

Roasted Coconut Brussels Sprouts

Brussels sprouts are often overcooked in boiling water, which causes them to have a very unpleasant odor. Roasting them is a great way to make sure they are perfect. Brussels sprouts are low in fat and sodium, and are a rich source of fiber, which makes them a smart choice when eating clean. They also have a cancer-fighting chemical in them called sulforaphane, which can be destroyed by boiling but stays intact when these vegetables are roasted.

Shopping tip Make sure you get unsweetened shredded coconut rather than the sweetened product. Or better yet, shred your own coconut meat from a fresh coconut to ensure there's no added sugar.

2 pounds Brussels sprouts, trimmed and cut in half

2 teaspoons coconut oil, melted

¼ cup unsweetened toasted shredded coconut

1. Preheat the oven to 400°F. Line a baking sheet with foil and set aside.
2. In a large bowl, toss the Brussels sprouts with the melted coconut oil until the vegetables are well coated.
3. Spread the Brussels sprouts on the prepared baking sheet in one layer and roast until they are tender and browned, about 20 to 30 minutes.
4. Serve topped with toasted coconut.

Serves 4. Prep time 10 minutes. Cook time 30 minutes.

Calories **117** / Calories from fat **25** / Total fat **2.7g** / Saturated fat **2.0g** / Sodium **57mg** / Carbs **21.4g** / Sugars **5.1g** / Protein **7.8g**

Whole-Wheat Farfalle with Mint Pesto

You can put this lovely, simple side dish on the table in less than half an hour and enjoy the compliments. Try adding any vegetables, such as cherry tomatoes, asparagus, or tender green beans, if you have them on hand. You can also use whatever pasta is available, but these pretty bowties are quite festive and unusual.

Cooking tip You can make the mint pesto up to a week ahead of time. Store it in the refrigerator in an airtight container until you need it.

½ cup fresh mint leaves

½ cup fresh basil leaves

4 tablespoons pecans

2 tablespoons grated Parmesan cheese

1 tablespoon fresh lemon juice

1 tablespoon olive oil

Freshly ground black pepper, to taste

8 ounces dry whole-wheat farfalle

1 cup chopped artichoke hearts, cooked
   or canned

1 cup chopped roasted red peppers

1. Fill a large pot with water and bring to a boil over high heat.
2. Meanwhile, in a food processor, combine the mint, basil, pecans, Parmesan cheese, lemon juice, olive oil, and pepper and pulse until a chunky paste forms, about 2 minutes. Scoop the pesto into a bowl and set aside.
3. When the water is boiling, cook the pasta to al dente, according to the package directions.
4. Drain the pasta and return it to the pot. Add the pesto, artichoke hearts, and red peppers.
5. Stir to combine and heat through, about 5 minutes.
6. Serve immediately.

Serves 4. Prep time 10 minutes. Cook time 20 minutes.

Calories **333** / Calories from fat **115** / Total fat **12.7g** / Saturated fat **3.0g** / Trans fat **0.0g** / Sodium **174mg** / Carbs **49.9g** / Sugars **0.8g** / Protein **14.0g**

FODMAP-free
Gluten-free
Low-fat
Nightshade-free
Vegan
Vegetarian

SIDE DISHES

Grilled Carrots with Dill

Carrots seem like such a humble vegetable, but when you put them on the grill they get an exotic, slightly smoky taste that combines beautifully with fresh dill. Try not to cut your carrot sticks too small or thin, because you might lose them through the grill grates.

Shopping tip Although you can get dried dill year round, the best time to get fresh dill is in the early spring and summer.

1 pound carrots, washed and cut into batons about 3 inches long and ½ inch thick

1 teaspoon olive oil

1 tablespoon chopped fresh dill

1 tablespoon fresh lemon juice

1. Preheat the barbecue to medium-high heat or preheat the broiler.
2. On the barbecue, grill the carrots until softened and lightly charred, turning frequently, about 10 minutes. Or in the oven, broil the carrots, turning once, until tender, about 8 minutes.
3. In a large bowl, combine the carrots with the remaining ingredients and toss.
4. Serve warm.

Serves 4. Prep time 5 minutes. Cook time 10 minutes.

Calories **59** / Calories from fat **14** / Total fat **1.5g** / Trans fat **0.0g** / Sodium **80mg** / Carbs **11.4g** / Sugars **5.5g** / Protein **1.2g**

Rosemary Roasted Beets

The texture and color of the beets are ideal next to a lean, perfectly grilled steak or baked fish such as halibut. Rosemary also combines well with both red meat and fish, but you don't need very much to create a strong flavor. Rosemary is a good source of iron, calcium, and vitamins A, B_6, and C, which means it can help detoxify the liver, reduce the risk of cancer, and help provide some relief from arthritis-associated pain.

Diet tip If you want this dish to be low-sodium, simply omit the pinch of salt at the end and add a little freshly ground black pepper instead.

4 cups peeled and quartered beets

1 tablespoon olive oil

1 tablespoon chopped fresh rosemary

Pinch of sea salt

1. Preheat the oven to 400°F. Line a baking tray with foil and set aside.
2. In a large bowl, toss the beets with the oil until the beets are coated.
3. Spread the beets on the prepared baking sheet and roast in the oven until the vegetables are tender and lightly browned, about 25 to 35 minutes.
4. Remove the beets from the oven and sprinkle with the rosemary.
5. Season with salt and serve hot.

Serves 4. Prep time 10 minutes. Cook time 25 to 35 minutes.

Calories **91** / Calories from fat **35** / Total fat **3.9g** / Saturated fat **0.6g** / Sodium **165mg** / Carbs **14.6g** / Sugars **9.2g** / Protein **2.2g**

Gluten-free
Low-fat
Low-sodium
Vegetarian
Vegan

SIDE DISHES

Potato Fennel Bake

Fennel bulbs look a little like very fat celery bunches but taste like licorice. This flavor can be strong when the fennel is raw, but mellows when the vegetable is roasted, as in this dish. Fennel is rich in B vitamins, vitamin C, iron, potassium, and manganese. It can support healthy digestion and reduce the risk of heart disease and cancer.

Shopping tip The fennel fronds should never have any flowering buds, because that means it is past maturity and could be slightly bitter. Fennel is best in the winter and early spring.

2 large Yukon gold potatoes, skin on, washed and thinly sliced
1 tablespoon olive oil
Freshly ground black pepper
1 medium fennel bulb, trimmed and thinly sliced

2 teaspoons chopped fresh thyme
2 garlic cloves, thinly sliced
Zest and juice of 1 lemon
1 cup low-sodium, fat-free vegetable stock

1. Preheat the oven to 350°F.
2. In a medium bowl, toss the potatoes with the oil and season lightly with the pepper.
3. In a 9-by-11-inch baking dish, make an even layer of half the fennel slices.
4. Top the fennel with half the potatoes, half the thyme, and half the garlic.
5. Repeat the layering to use up all the fennel, potatoes, thyme, and garlic.
6. Sprinkle the casserole with lemon zest and juice.
7. Pour in the vegetable stock and cover the dish with foil.
8. Bake until the vegetables are very tender, about 45 minutes.
9. Remove the foil and bake for 5 more minutes to brown the potatoes.
10. Serve immediately.

Serves 4. Prep time 15 minutes. Cook time 50 minutes.

Calories **168** / Calories from fat **35** / Total fat **3.9g** / Saturated fat **0.6g** / Trans fat **0.0g** / Sodium **81mg** / Carbs **33.9g** / Sugars **1.8g** / Protein **4.2g**

Barley Kale Risotto

Risotto is usually prepared with a short- or medium-grain rice such as arborio, but it can also be prepared with most grains. Barley has a delightful chewy texture and nutty flavor, and it is an excellent source of fiber. Barley is also rich in manganese, selenium, copper, and vitamin B_1. It can help protect against heart disease, type 2 diabetes, and breast cancer.

Shopping tip You can usually find hulled barley in the bulk sections of major grocery stores. Make sure the containers of barley are tightly covered so there is no moisture, and that your grocery store has a rotation policy to ensure the freshness of the product.

1 medium butternut squash, peeled, seeded, and cut into ½ inch cubes

2 teaspoons olive oil, divided

Pinch of freshly ground black pepper

½ small sweet onion, peeled and finely chopped

1 teaspoon minced garlic

1 cup hulled barley, rinsed

4 cups chopped kale

2 tablespoons pine nuts

2 tablespoons chopped fresh thyme

1. Preheat the oven to 375°F. Line a baking sheet with foil.
2. Toss the squash with 1 teaspoon of the oil and the pepper.
3. Spread the squash on the prepared baking sheet and roast in the oven until the squash is tender and lightly browned, stirring several times, about 35 minutes.
4. While the squash is roasting, fill a medium saucepan with about 5 cups of water and bring to a boil.
5. Reduce the heat to keep the water warm but not simmering.
6. In a large saucepan over medium heat, add the remaining teaspoon of oil and sauté the onion and garlic in the oil until softened, about 3 minutes.
7. Add the barley and sauté, stirring, for about 2 minutes.
8. Add one cup of the hot water to the barley and stir until the water is absorbed.

continued ➤

9. Repeat until you have added 3 cups of hot water to the barley.
10. Add the kale and stir until the kale is wilted and the water is absorbed.
11. Add more water, a small amount at a time, stirring often, until the barley is cooked through and tender.
12. Stir in the roasted squash and the pine nuts.
13. Serve the risotto topped with thyme.

Serves 4. Prep time 10 minutes. Cook time 1 hour.

Calories **323** / Calories from fat **75** / Total fat **8.3g** / Saturated fat **0.8g** / Trans fat **0.0g** / Sodium **37mg** / Carbs **58.5g** / Sugars **6.2g** / Protein **10.1g**

Tomato-Topped Spaghetti Squash

Gluten-free
Low-fat
Low-sodium
Nightshade-free
Vegetarian

SIDE DISHES

The pasta-like appearance of cooked spaghetti squash makes it popular for vegan, vegetarian, and gluten-free dishes. The texture is softer than pasta, so do not over-cook this vegetable if you want a firmer "noodle" for the side dish. You can also use a Clean Eating marinara sauce instead of fresh tomatoes to top the squash.

Shopping tip When picking your spaghetti squash, look for one with a firm dry stem because the stem can keep bacteria out of the inside of the squash.

1 spaghetti squash, cut in half lengthwise

1 tablespoon olive oil

Sea salt

Freshly ground black pepper

2 tomatoes, chopped

2 tablespoons chopped green onion

1 tablespoon chopped fresh basil or 3 teaspoons dried basil

3 tablespoons Parmesan cheese

1. Preheat oven to 350°F.
2. Line a baking tray with foil.
3. Scoop the seeds out of the squash and drizzle the cut sides with the olive oil.
4. Season the cut sides lightly with salt and pepper and lay the squash halves cut-side down on the baking sheet.
5. Bake the squash until it is tender, about 45 minutes. Let the squash cool on the tray for 10 minutes.
6. While the squash is baking, combine the tomatoes, green onion, and basil in a small bowl; set aside.
7. Use a fork to shred the squash strands into a medium bowl.
8. Top the shredded squash with the tomato mixture and Parmesan cheese and serve immediately.

Serves 2. Prep time 10 minutes. Cook time 45 minutes.

Calories **129** / Calories from fat **47** / Total fat **5.2g** / Saturated fat **1.6g** / Sodium **223mg** / Carbs **19.5g** / Sugars **3.3g** / Protein **4.8g**

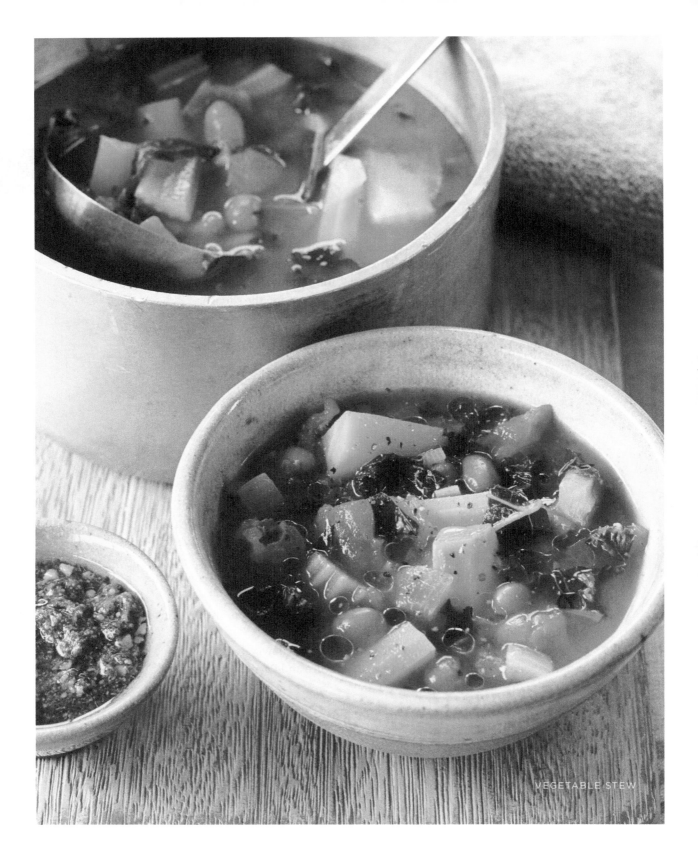

VEGETABLE STEW

CHAPTER TEN

Vegetarian Entrées

Bean Tostadas

Tostada is "toasted" in Spanish; this dish is a toasted tortilla topped with an array of delicious toppings. You can use any tortilla—corn, multigrain, or even gluten-free—for this dish. The jalapeño peppers in this recipe give a nice heat, which can be kicked up by using chipotle or even habañero peppers instead. Make sure you wash your hands thoroughly after handling the hot peppers, because the juices can severely irritate any mucus membranes they come in contact with.

Diet tip This recipe can easily be made gluten-free by using gluten-free tortillas instead of whole-wheat. Leave out the feta cheese and it's vegan.

Eight 6-inch whole-wheat tortillas
Nonstick cooking spray
3 cups canned sodium-free black beans, drained and rinsed
1 small sweet onion, peeled and coarsely chopped
1 red bell pepper, seeded and diced

2 jalapeño peppers, seeded and coarsely chopped
1 teaspoon ground cumin
4 tablespoons water
4 teaspoons chopped fresh cilantro
¼ cup crumbled low-sodium feta
1 large tomato, diced
1 cup shredded romaine lettuce

1. Preheat the oven to 400°F.
2. On two baking sheets, toast the tortillas in the oven until crisp, about 5 minutes.
3. Remove the tortillas from the baking sheets and set aside.
4. Lightly coat the baking sheets with cooking spray and spread the beans, onion, red pepper, and jalapeño peppers evenly on the sheets; roast the mixture in the oven for about 10 minutes.
5. In a food processor, combine the roasted beans and vegetables with the cumin and water and pulse until coarsely chopped.
6. On each tortilla, spread an equal amount of the bean mixture and sprinkle with the cilantro and feta.

7. Top each with the tomato and shredded lettuce.
8. Serve two tostadas per person.

Serves 4. Prep time 10 minutes. Cook time 15 minutes.

Calories **250** / Calories from fat **30** / Total fat **3.3g** / Saturated fat **0.7g** / Trans fat **0.0g** /
Sodium **554mg** / Carbs **55.4g** / Sugars **2.4g** / Protein **10.6g**

Grilled Portobello Burgers with Goat Cheese

These large, meaty mushrooms are a favorite of many vegetarians. So why not use them as burger patties? Portobello mushrooms can be up to four inches in diameter, so they fit perfectly on most buns. They are a good source of fiber, protein, vitamin D, and potassium, and are low in calories and fat.

Cooking tip Make sure to brush your mushrooms evenly with oil, rather than tossing them, because these mushrooms can soak up the oil unevenly, creating dry sections when you grill them.

4 large Portobello mushroom caps, each about 4 inches in diameter

1 tablespoon olive oil

1 large red onion, cut into ¼-inch-thick slices

2 tablespoons balsamic vinegar

4 ciabatta buns, split

4 tablespoons crumbled goat cheese

1 large tomato, cut into ¼-inch-thick slices

1 cup shredded Boston lettuce

1. Preheat a barbecue to medium-high or preheat the broiler.
2. Brush the mushroom caps with the oil.
3. In a large bowl, combine the mushroom caps with the onion and toss with the balsamic vinegar.
4. On the barbecue, grill the mushroom caps and onion until they are tender, about 5 minutes per side. Or if using the oven, place the caps on a baking tray and broil until the mushrooms and onions are tender, about 5 minutes.
5. Remove from the heat and set aside on a plate.
6. Place the buns on the barbecue, cut-side down, and toast for about 1 minute. Or place them under the broiler, cut-side up, and broil for about 30 seconds.
7. Spread the goat cheese on the top bun halves.
8. Place a mushroom on each bun bottom and top with the onions.

9. Place a tomato slice on the onions and ¼ cup of the shredded lettuce for each bun.

10. Top with the top bun halves and serve.

Serves 4. Prep time 5 minutes. Cook time 15 minutes.

Calories **338** / Calories from fat **105** / Total fat **11.7g** / Saturated fat **5.0g** / Trans fat **0.0g** / Sodium **494mg** / Carbs **42.1g** / Sugars **5.9g** / Protein **14.8g**

Vegetable Stew

This recipe is only a guideline for the finished dish, because you can add any combination of vegetables and still have a delicious stew. The combination of vegetables in the ingredients provide an array of colors, textures, and tastes, giving you a complete culinary and nutrition experience in one bowl. Eating many different colors of produce means you are getting a full range of antioxidants and nutrients.

1 teaspoon olive oil

1 small sweet onion, peeled and chopped

1 teaspoon minced garlic

½ teaspoon ground cumin

½ teaspoon ground coriander

1 red bell pepper, seeded and chopped

2 large carrots, peeled and chopped

2 cups fat-free, low-sodium vegetable stock

2 large tomatoes, chopped

½ cup canned sodium-free white kidney
    beans, rinsed and drained

1 teaspoon fresh lemon juice

1 cup chopped kale

Pinch of crushed red pepper flakes

Freshly ground black pepper, to taste

1. In a large pot over medium heat, heat the oil and sauté the onion and garlic until softened, about 3 minutes.
2. Add the cumin, and coriander, and stir to coat, about 1 minute.
3. Add the red pepper and carrots and sauté for 5 minutes.
4. Stir in the vegetable stock, tomatoes, and kidney beans.
5. Bring the stew to a boil and then reduce the heat to low.
6. Simmer the stew until the vegetables are tender, stirring often, about 15 to 17 minutes.
7. Add the lemon juice and kale and heat until the kale is wilted, about 3 minutes.
8. Stir in the red pepper flakes and pepper.
9. Serve.

Serves 4. Prep time 15 minutes. Cook time 30 minutes.

Calories **101** / Calories from fat **16** / Total fat **1.8g** / Saturated fat **0.0g** / Trans fat **0.0g** / Sodium **63mg** / Carbs **17.7g** / Sugars **7.2g** / Protein **4.4g**

Simple Colcannon

Gluten-free
Low-fat
Vegan
Vegetarian

VEGETARIAN
ENTRÉES

Colcannon is a traditional Irish dish of cabbage and mashed potatoes with a history dating back hundreds of years. If you want to add a couple of cups of shredded green cabbage along with (or instead of) the kale, you will be in good culinary company, since that is the more traditional ingredient. Simply sauté the cabbage until it is tender, about ten minutes, before adding the kale.

Nutrition tip Let your chopped kale sit for about five minutes before cooking. This can increase the phytonutrient benefits because the "wounded" leaves produce anti-oxidants to repair the damage.

6 large russet potatoes, peeled and
     chopped into ½-inch chunks
1 teaspoon olive oil
1 small sweet onion, peeled and diced
3 teaspoons minced garlic

6 cups chopped kale
1 cup almond milk
Pinch of sea salt
Pinch of freshly ground black pepper

1. Bring a large pot of water to a boil over medium-high heat, and add the potatoes.
2. Boil until the potatoes are tender, about 15 minutes.
3. Drain and rinse the potatoes, and transfer them to a large bowl. Set aside.
4. In a large skillet over medium-high heat, heat the oil and sauté the onion and garlic until softened, about 3 minutes.
5. Add the kale and sauté until it is wilted, about 3 minutes.
6. Mash the potatoes with the almond milk, salt, and pepper until smooth.
7. Add the kale mixture to the mashed potatoes and stir until well combined.
8. Serve warm.

Serves 4. Prep time 15 minutes. Cook time 25 minutes.

Calories **370** / Calories from fat **22** / Total fat **2.4g** / Saturated fat **0.0g** / Trans fat **0.0g** / Sodium **189mg** / Carbs **77.4g** / Sugars **4.0g** / Protein **11.4g**

Baked Broccoli Rice Cakes

These are like golden savory muffins rather than cakes. Broccoli and cheese is a classic combination that works well with the rice in this dish. Broccoli is a vegetable you just can't eat often enough, because it is packed with nutrients and antioxidants. Broccoli can help boost the immune system and support healthy bones, as well.

Cooking tip Fresh broccoli can be stored in the refrigerator in a sealed plastic bag for as long as ten days if you leave it on the stalk and don't wash it until you're ready to cook it. If you cut it into florets before storing, the vitamin C content will start to diminish after a few days.

Nonstick cooking spray

2 cups chopped broccoli florets

2 cups cooked brown rice

¼ cup plain Greek yogurt

2 eggs, lightly beaten

½ cup grated sharp Cheddar cheese

¼ teaspoon ground nutmeg

Freshly ground black pepper

1. Preheat the oven to 350°F. Lightly coat 8 muffin cups with cooking spray and set aside.
2. Fill a medium saucepan with water and bring to a boil over medium-high heat.
3. Add the broccoli to the boiling water and blanch until it is tender-crisp, about 3 minutes. Drain the broccoli.
4. In a large bowl, combine the broccoli with the rice, yogurt, eggs, cheese, and nutmeg, and season with pepper to taste.
5. Portion the broccoli mixture evenly among the muffin cups and bake until golden, about 20 minutes.
6. Remove the cakes from the oven and let them stand for 5 minutes. Run a knife around the edges to loosen.
7. Serve two cakes per person with a green salad.

Serves 4. Prep time 10 minutes. Cook time 25 minutes.

Calories **461** / Calories from fat **93** / Total fat **10.3g** / Saturated fat **4.6g** / Trans fat **0.0g** / Sodium **142mg** / Carbs **76.3g** / Sugars **1.6g** / Protein **15.9g**

Market Quinoa Skillet

This packed skillet is a filling and satisfying choice on cold winter evenings when you crave comfort food. The quinoa provides bulk, along with many important nutrients, and is incredibly easy to prepare.

Diet tip Creating a vegan meal is as simple as leaving out the feta cheese or adding a favorite vegan cheese product in its place.

2 cups fat-free, low-sodium
　　vegetable stock
1 cup uncooked quinoa, rinsed and drained
1 teaspoon olive oil
2 teaspoons minced garlic
2 cups fresh corn kernels
2 cups chopped green beans, cut into
　　1-inch pieces
½ large zucchini, cut in half lengthwise and
　　thinly sliced into half disks

1 red bell pepper, seeded and sliced
　　into thin strips
2 green onions, thinly sliced
2 ripe tomatoes, chopped
½ cup crumbled low-sodium feta cheese
3 teaspoons chopped fresh basil
2 tablespoons fresh lemon juice
2 teaspoons lemon zest
Pinch of freshly ground black pepper

1. In a medium saucepan over medium heat, bring the vegetable stock to a boil and then add the quinoa.
2. Cover and reduce the heat to low.
3. Cook until the quinoa has absorbed all the stock, about 15 minutes.
4. Remove the quinoa from the heat and let it cool slightly.
5. In a large skillet over medium-high heat, heat the oil and sauté the garlic until softened, about 1 minute.
6. Add the corn, green beans, zucchini, red pepper, and green onions, and sauté until the vegetables are tender-crisp, about 5 minutes.
7. Add the quinoa and the remaining ingredients. Stir to combine.
8. Serve warm or cold.

Serves 4. Prep time 15 minutes. Cook time 30 minutes.

Calories **302** / Calories from fat **64** / Total fat **7.1g** / Saturated fat **2.1g** / Trans fat **0.0g** / Sodium **606mg** / Carbs **51.9g** / Sugars **7.4g** / Protein **16.2g**

Broccolini Sauté

Broccolini looks like baby broccoli, but it is actually a hybrid of Chinese and regular broccoli, and tastes more like asparagus than broccoli. It has long, slender stalks and tight green buds that do not need much cooking time. Broccolini has all the health benefits of broccoli, as well, making this dish a wonderfully nutritious, light dinner for any vegetarian or vegan.

Nutrition tip This delicate vegetable is a naturally occurring hybrid rather than a genetically modified one.

3 teaspoons olive oil

4 cups chopped broccolini
(about 3 bunches)

3 green onions, chopped

4 roasted garlic cloves, sliced or chopped (see page 190)

½ teaspoon freshly ground black pepper

¼ teaspoon crushed red pepper flakes

3 cups baby spinach

¼ cup chopped fresh parsley

Zest and juice of 1 lemon

1. In a large skillet over medium heat, heat the oil and sauté the broccolini, green onions, and roasted garlic until the broccolini is bright green but still crisp, about 5 minutes.
2. Add the black pepper and red pepper flakes and stir to combine.
3. Add the spinach, parsley, and lemon zest and sauté until the spinach is wilted, about 3 minutes.
4. Add the lemon juice to the skillet and stir.
5. Serve immediately.

Serves 4. Prep time 10 minutes. Cook time 10 minutes.

Calories **81** / Calories from fat **33** / Total fat **3.7g** / Saturated fat **0.5g** / Trans fat **0.0g** / Sodium **47mg** / Carbs **8.2g** / Sugars **2.5g** / Protein **4.2g**

Red Lentil Coconut Curry

Gluten-free
Low-sodium
Vegan
Vegetarian

VEGETARIAN
ENTRÉES

Curry is a staple dish in vegetarian cuisine because the grains and root vegetables in a typical curry really soak up the seasonings. Coconut is also a very popular addition in all forms, such as shredded meat, milk, and even coconut water as in this recipe. Coconut water is the liquid that is taken from young coconuts, and is not to be confused with coconut milk, which is made from squeezing the liquid out of the meat.

Nutrition tip Coconut water is fat free, cholesterol free, low fat, and low sodium. It also has four times the amount of potassium as bananas, so it's a great recovery drink after a workout. You can find this super drink in most health food stores or in the organic sections of major grocery stores.

1 tablespoon coconut oil

1 small sweet onion, peeled and diced

2 teaspoons minced garlic

2 medium carrots, peeled and diced

1 sweet potato, peeled and diced

2 teaspoons grated fresh ginger

1 tablespoon curry powder

3 large ripe tomatoes, diced

2 cups fat-free, low-sodium
    vegetable stock

1 cup coconut water

1 cup dried red lentils, rinsed and
    picked through

1 cup finely julienned spinach

1. In a large pot over medium heat, heat the coconut oil and sauté the onion and garlic until softened, about 3 minutes.
2. Add the carrots and sweet potato and sauté for 10 more minutes, stirring often.
3. Add the remaining ingredients except the spinach and stir to combine.
4. Bring the mixture to a boil and then reduce the heat to low.
5. Simmer the curry until most of the liquid is absorbed and the lentils and vegetables are tender, about 30 minutes.
6. Stir in the spinach and let the curry stand for about 10 minutes.
7. Serve plain or over rice.

Serves 6. Prep time 15 minutes. Cook time 45 minutes.

Calories **288** / Calories from fat **41** / Total fat **4.6g** / Saturated fat **3.1g** / Trans fat **0.0g** /
Sodium **60mg** / Carbs **34.1g** / Sugars **8.7g** / Protein **16.2g**

Healthy Vegetable Chili

Making a spectacular chili is a mark of honor among many serious cooks, and there are serious competitions geared around this simple dish. This version is more than just a combination of beans, tomato, and spices; it is also packed with a nice assortment of healthy vegetables. If you want to substitute different vegetables, don't feel like you have to stick to the recipe. Chili is very accommodating of most ingredient choices.

Nutrition tip Chili powder is produced from dried chili peppers, and it can be mildly hot or it can sear your throat, depending on what chili pepper is used. Chili peppers contain a substance called capsaicin that creates this distinctive heat. It also can be an effective treatment for pain associated with osteoarthritis.

2 tablespoons olive oil

1 large sweet onion, peeled and finely chopped

3 teaspoons minced garlic

2 cups chopped button mushrooms

2 large carrots, peeled and diced

1 large red bell pepper, seeded and diced

1 large zucchini, diced

1 jalapeño pepper, seeded and chopped

¼ cup chili powder

1 tablespoon ground cumin

1 tablespoon dried oregano

1 teaspoon crushed red pepper flakes

4 large tomatoes, chopped

One 6-ounce can sodium-free tomato paste

1 cup fat-free, low-sodium vegetable stock

2 cups black beans, rinsed and drained

2 cups red kidney beans, rinsed and drained

2 cups navy beans, rinsed and drained

1. In a large pot over medium-high heat, heat the olive oil and sauté the onion, garlic, and mushrooms until softened, about 3 minutes.
2. Add the carrots, red bell pepper, and zucchini and sauté for an additional 8 minutes.
3. Add the remaining ingredients and stir to combine well.
4. Bring the chili to a boil and then reduce the heat to low.

5. Simmer the vegetables until they are fork tender and the flavors have mellowed, about 45 minutes.
6. Remove the chili from the heat and let it stand for about 10 minutes before serving.

Serves 12. Prep time 15 minutes. Cook time 1 hour.

Calories **408** / Calories from fat **51** / Total fat **5.7g** / Saturated fat **1.7g** / Trans fat **0.0g** / Sodium **54mg** / Carbs **69.1g** / Sugars **7.2g** / Protein **23.8g**

Lentil Barley Burgers

The complexity of flavor found in these veggie burgers might surprise you if you are used to the bland, processed versions. Red lentils are the base for these burgers, but you can also use green, yellow, or brown lentils. The color will change and the flavor will also slightly change, because red lentils are the sweetest and nuttiest variety.

Shopping tip You can either cook your own lentils (they cook much faster than beans) or buy an organic, sodium-free cooked product to save time.

3 teaspoons olive oil, divided

½ small sweet onion, chopped

3 tablespoons grated carrot

1 teaspoon minced garlic

1 teaspoon ground cumin

1 teaspoon dried oregano

Pinch of chili powder

Pinch of salt

½ cup cooked lentils, rinsed and drained

½ cup cooked pearl barley

¼ cup panko breadcrumbs

3 tablespoons chopped fresh parsley

1 egg white

1 egg

1 large mango, peeled, pitted, and diced

1. In a medium skillet over medium heat, heat 1 teaspoon of the olive oil and sauté the onion, carrot, and garlic until the vegetables are softened.
2. Add the cumin, oregano, chili powder, and salt and stir to combine. Remove from the heat.
3. In a large mixing bowl, combine the onion mixture with the remaining ingredients, except for the mango.
4. Stir until the mixture holds together well, adding more panko if the mixture is too wet.
5. Cover the burger mixture and refrigerate until firm, about 1 hour.
6. Divide the burger mixture into four portions, and press them into four ½-inch-thick patties.

7. In a large skillet over medium-high heat, heat the remaining 2 teaspoons of olive oil and cook the patties until both sides are golden brown, about 3 minutes per side.
8. Serve topped with mango.

Serves 4. Prep time 15 minutes. Cook time 11 minutes.

Calories **355** / Calories from fat **89** / Total fat **9.9g** / Saturated fat **2.3g** / Trans fat **0.0g** / Sodium **147mg** / Carbs **49.9g** / Sugars **10.0g** / Protein **17.6g**

Mushroom Cashew Rice

The cashews in this hearty rice dish provide an interesting crunch and richness that is very pleasing to the palate. Cashews are heart-healthy, can help reduce the risk of cancer, and promote bone health. Despite the bad reputation nuts usually have because of their fat content, cashews actually support weight loss as well. They contain healthy fats and are an energy-dense choice for dieters.

Shopping tip When buying cashews, especially in bulk, it is important to smell them to make sure they aren't rancid. Cashews can be stored in the refrigerator in a sealed container for up to six months.

1 tablespoon olive oil

3 celery stalks, chopped

½ small sweet onion, peeled and chopped

2 teaspoons minced garlic

1 cup sliced button mushrooms

2 cups uncooked brown basmati rice

3½ cups fat-free, low-sodium vegetable stock

Freshly ground black pepper

½ cup chopped cashews

1. In a large saucepan over medium-high heat, heat the oil and sauté the celery, onion, garlic, and mushrooms until they are softened.
2. Add the rice and sauté for an additional minute.
3. Add the stock and bring to a boil, then reduce the heat to low and cover the pot.
4. Simmer the rice until the liquid is absorbed and the rice is tender, about 35 to 40 minutes.
5. Season with pepper to taste.
6. Top with cashews and serve.

Serves 6. Prep time 10 minutes. Cook time 15 minutes.

Calories **341** / Calories from fat **80** / Total fat **8.9g** / Saturated fat **1.7g** / Trans fat **0.0g** / Sodium **458mg** / Carbs **51.1g** / Sugars **1.7g** / Protein **9.5g**

Lemon Artichoke Pesto with Zucchini Noodles

This is a truly gorgeous example of everything that is wonderful about vegetarian cuisine. It is colorful, fresh, and packed with flavor. The artichokes add a richness and bulk to the pesto and finished dish, as well as some important health benefits. Artichokes are extremely high in antioxidants, which means they are super disease fighters. Artichokes can cut your risk of cancer, reduce cholesterol, and support effective liver function.

Leftovers tip You might not use up all the pesto in this recipe. Spoon the extra into ice cube trays, cover the whole tray in plastic wrap, and freeze it for up to six months.

1 cup chopped artichoke hearts

½ cup packed fresh basil leaves

½ cup chopped pecan halves

2 teaspoons minced garlic

Zest and juice of 1 lemon

Pinch of freshly ground black pepper

¼ cup olive oil

2 large zucchini, julienned

2 cups cherry tomatoes, halved

Pinch of crushed red pepper flakes

1. In a food processor, combine half the artichoke hearts with the basil, pecans, garlic, lemon zest, lemon juice, and black pepper; pulse until very finely chopped.
2. Add the olive oil and pulse until blended.
3. In a large bowl, toss the zucchini "noodles" with the remaining artichoke hearts, cherry tomatoes, and red pepper flakes until well mixed.
4. Add the pesto by tablespoons until you have the desired flavor and texture.
5. Store any leftover pesto in a sealed container in the refrigerator for up to 2 weeks.
6. Serve immediately.

Serves 4. Prep time 30 minutes.

Calories **259** / Calories from fat **203** / Total fat **22.6g** / Saturated fat **2.7g** / Trans Fat **0.0g** / Sodium **106mg** / Carbs **14.1g** / Sugars **5.4g** / Protein **5.4g**

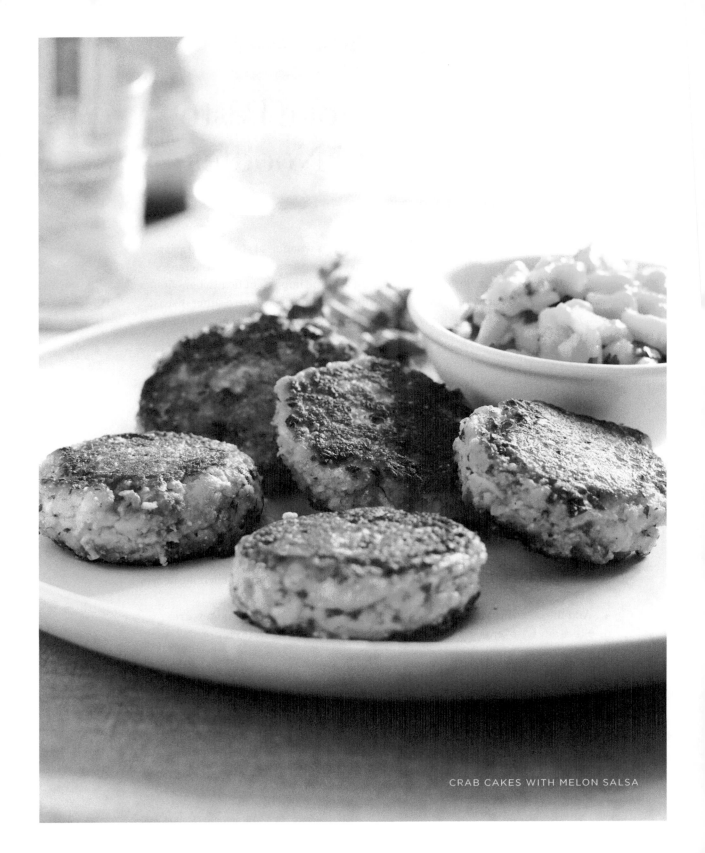

CRAB CAKES WITH MELON SALSA

CHAPTER ELEVEN

Seafood

Cod with Cucumber Mint Sauce

This dish is spring on a plate—snowy, tender fish topped with delicate pastel green cucumber and cool mint. It is a delight to the taste and light on the stomach. Mint is high in vitamins A and C, and is also a good source of copper, calcium, potassium, and magnesium. It can stimulate digestion, boost the immune system, and cleanse the blood.

Shopping tip Whenever possible, buy Pacific cod because the Atlantic cod population is diminishing. This white fish should be firm and slightly springy to the touch with a very mild fish scent.

Nonstick cooking spray

Four 5-ounce cod fillets

Sea salt

Freshly ground black pepper

4 tablespoons fat-free plain Greek yogurt

¼ English cucumber, grated, liquid squeezed out

2 teaspoons chopped fresh mint

2 tablespoons chopped green onion

1. In a large skillet over medium-high heat, add a light coat of cooking spray.
2. Season the fish with salt and pepper to taste and pan fry the fish in the skillet, turning once, until it is just cooked through, about 4 minutes per side. Remove the fish from the heat and transfer the fillets to individual plates.
3. In a small bowl, stir together the yogurt, cucumber, mint, and green onion until well mixed.
4. Serve the fish topped with the yogurt sauce.

Serves 4. Prep time 10 minutes. Cook time 8 minutes.

Calories **127** / Calories from fat **12** / Total fat **1.3g** / Saturated fat **0.0g** / Trans fat **0.0g** / Sodium **96mg** / Carbs **1.0g** / Sugar **0.0g** / Protein **27.0g**

Kale Quinoa Topped with Halibut

This recipe produces a side dish and main course in one. Kale is one of those super greens that are now available in most grocery stores and markets. It is rich in calcium, beta-carotene, chlorophyll, and vitamins A, C, and K. Kale can support a healthy digestive system, improve eyesight, and reduce the risk of heart disease, cancer, and type 2 diabetes.

Shopping tip Fresh halibut is usually best between March and November. If you buy frozen halibut, it takes about one-third less cooking time than fresh. Cook the fish after it has thawed.

1 cup uncooked quinoa, rinsed

2 cups water

Nonstick cooking spray

½ small sweet onion, peeled and chopped

1 cup diced cooked sweet potato

2 cups chopped kale

Four 4-ounce halibut fillets

Sea salt

Freshly ground black pepper

1. In a medium saucepan, combine the quinoa and water.
2. Bring the quinoa to a boil over medium-high heat and then reduce the heat to low so the liquid simmers.
3. Cover and cook the quinoa until all the liquid is absorbed, about 15 minutes.
4. Transfer the quinoa to a large bowl and set aside.
5. In a large nonstick skillet, add a light coat of cooking spray and heat over medium-high heat.
6. Add the onion and sauté until it is softened, about 3 minutes.
7. Stir in the cooked sweet potato and sauté until heated through, about 5 minutes.
8. Add the kale and stir until it is wilted, about 3 minutes.
9. Add the quinoa mixture to the kale and stir to mix well.

continued ➤

SEAFOOD

10. Preheat the oven to broil.
11. Place the halibut on a small baking sheet and season with salt and pepper to taste.
12. Broil the fish, turning once, until the fish flakes when pressed with a fork, about 4 minutes per side.
13. Serve the fish over the quinoa.

Serves 4. Prep time 10 minutes. Cook time 35 minutes.

Calories **401** / Calories from fat **87** / Total fat **9.6g** / Saturated fat **1.3g** / Trans fat **0.0g** / Sodium **111mg** / Carbs **39.8g** / Sugars **4.4g** / Protein **38.4g**

Ginger Salmon in Foil Packets

This is similar to cooking fish "en papillote" (in parchment), so go ahead and create parchment-paper packets if you are familiar with that culinary technique. This dish has some definite Asian flavors, using cut vegetables, sesame, and ginger.

Nutrition tip Bean sprouts are crunchy and sweet, but they are also very heart-friendly due to their high potassium and vitamin K content. Bean sprouts are also a good source of fiber, which can help lower cholesterol levels.

4 cups bean sprouts
1 large red bell pepper, seeded and thinly sliced into strips
1 cup snow peas, stringed and halved
Four 4-ounce salmon fillets, skin removed
¼ cup fat-free, low-sodium vegetable stock

2 teaspoons grated fresh ginger
1 green onion, chopped finely
½ teaspoon minced garlic
1 teaspoon sesame oil
2 tablespoons sesame seeds

1. Preheat the oven to 400°F. Cut four pieces of foil, each about 12 inches square.
2. Evenly divide the bean sprouts, red pepper, and snow peas into quarters and place onto the middle of each piece of foil.
3. Place a salmon fillet on top of each pile of vegetables.
4. In a small bowl, stir together the vegetable stock, ginger, green onion, garlic, and oil until well mixed.
5. Drizzle the sauce evenly over the salmon.
6. Fold the foil up into sealed packets and place them on a baking sheet.
7. Bake until the fish flakes when pressed with a fork, about 20 minutes.
8. Remove the salmon and vegetables from the foil and top each serving with sesame seeds.

Serves 4. Prep time 10 minutes. Cook time 20 minutes.

Calories **276** / Calories from fat **104** / Total fat **11.6g** / Saturated fat **1.6g** / Trans fat **0.0g** / Sodium **91mg** / Carbs **14.9g** / Sugars **3.8g** / Protein **32.6g**

Crab Cakes with Melon Salsa

This salsa elevates what is a very nice dish to something truly special. Crab and fruit are a naturally good combination, especially with the addition of a little acid such as lemon juice. Cantaloupe and watermelon are very well known for their health benefits, but the often underused honeydew is also a nutritional prize. It is high in fiber, potassium, and vitamins B_6 and C.

Shopping tip When picking honeydew, sniff the melon to make sure it is ripe. You will be able to smell the flesh right through the pale, creamy skin if it is ready to eat.

For the salsa:
1 cup finely diced honeydew
½ cup finely diced watermelon
½ cup finely diced cantaloupe
1 green onion, finely chopped
2 tablespoons fresh lemon juice
Pinch of sea salt

For the crab cakes:
1 pound cooked lump crabmeat, drained
    and picked over
¼ cup whole-wheat panko breadcrumbs
2 teaspoons Dijon mustard
2 green onions, finely chopped
1 tablespoon chopped fresh parsley
1 teaspoon freshly grated lemon zest
1 teaspoon smoked paprika
2 egg whites
4 tablespoons whole-wheat flour
Nonstick cooking spray

To make the salsa:
1. In a medium bowl, combine all the salsa ingredients and mix well.
2. Store the salsa in a sealed container in the refrigerator until serving the crab cakes.

To make the crab cakes:
1. In a large bowl, combine the crabmeat, panko, mustard, green onions, parsley, lemon zest, paprika, and egg whites and mix very well.

2. Divide the crab mixture into 8 equal portions and form each portion into a patty about 1 inch thick.
3. Transfer the crab cakes to a plate, cover, and chill them in the refrigerator for at least an hour or overnight to firm up.
4. Put the flour on a plate and dredge the chilled crab cakes in the flour until they are lightly coated.
5. In a large skillet over medium heat, add a light coat of cooking spray and cook the crab cakes until they are golden brown, turning once, about 5 minutes per side.
6. Serve the crab cakes with the salsa.

Serves 4. Prep time 30 minutes. Cook time 10 minutes.

Calories **216** / Calories from fat **26** / Total fat **2.9g** / Trans fat **0.0g** / Sodium **554mg** / Carbs **36.4g** / Sugars **7.2g** / Protein **27.4g**

Spicy Lime Tilapia

Tilapia is a very popular fish because it is inexpensive and has a pleasant, mild taste that combines well with many other ingredients. Tilapia is rich in protein and omega-3 fatty acids, which are considered to be very heart-friendly. Because most tilapia is farmed, try to limit your consumption to one meal a week even though the fish is classified as a low-mercury fish. Farmed fish can sometimes have a high concentration of antibiotics, pesticides, and other contaminants such as PCBs. Fish is still considered to be a clean eating choice, but wild caught is preferred.

Leftovers tip This spicy fish is fabulous cold and tucked into a pita, or wrapped in a tortilla the next day with a little shredded spinach.

Four 6-ounce tilapia fillets

1 teaspoon chili powder

1 teaspoon garlic powder

½ teaspoon freshly ground black pepper

¼ teaspoon cayenne pepper

Nonstick olive oil cooking spray

Juice of 1 lime

1. Preheat the oven to 450°F. Line a baking sheet with foil and set aside. Pat the fish fillets dry with paper towels and place them on the prepared baking sheet. Set aside.
2. In a small bowl, stir together the chili and garlic powders, pepper, and cayenne until well mixed.
3. Sprinkle half of the spice mixture evenly over the fish and use your fingertips to lightly rub it in.
4. Spray a little olive oil over the fish and then sprinkle half of the lime juice over the fillets.
5. Flip the fish fillets over and repeat steps 3 and 4 on the other sides.
6. Bake in the oven until the fish flakes, about 8 minutes.

Serves 4. Prep time 15 minutes. Cook time 8 minutes.

Calories **145** / Calories from fat **15** / Total fat **1.7g** / Saturated fat **0.7g** / Trans fat **0.0g** / Sodium **67mg** / Carbs **1.1g** / Sugar **0.0g** / Protein **31.9g**

Salmon with Herbed Yogurt Sauce

Salmon is often found in clean eating plans because it is rich in omega-3 fatty acids, calcium, selenium, and vitamins A, B, and D. Salmon is very heart-smart, helps prevent Alzheimer's disease, and can boost your metabolism. Salmon can also support healthy hair, glowing skin, and clear eyes.

Nutrition tip Greek yogurt is packed with gut-friendly probiotics, which are beneficial bacteria. Probiotics help support a healthy immune system and stabilize the balance of flora in your digestive tract.

½ cup plain Greek yogurt

2 tablespoons fresh lime juice

1 tablespoon chopped fresh cilantro

1 teaspoon chopped fresh dill

1 teaspoon chopped fresh thyme

Freshly ground black pepper

Nonstick olive oil cooking spray

Four 6-ounce salmon fillets, skinned

1. In a small bowl, stir together the yogurt, lime juice, cilantro, dill, and thyme and then season with pepper to taste.
2. Store the sauce in a sealed container in the refrigerator until you are ready to serve the salmon; the sauce will keep for up to 2 days.
3. In a large skillet over medium-high heat, add a light coat of olive oil spray.
4. Season the salmon with pepper to taste and cook in the preheated skillet, turning once, until the fish flakes when pressed, about 4 minutes per side.
5. Serve with the herbed yogurt sauce.

Serves 4. Prep time 5 minutes. Cook time 8 minutes.

Calories **256** / Calories from fat **105** / Total fat **11.7g** / Saturated fat **2.3g** / Trans fat **0.0g** / Sodium **86mg** / Carbs **3.3g** / Sugars **1.5g** / Protein **35.7g**

Lemon Tuna Patties

Canned tuna becomes a sophisticated, citrusy patty in this dish that also has a generous herb flavoring. Lemon is very high in limonene and vitamin C, and is a good source of citric acid, calcium, vitamin A, and potassium. It is a great detoxifier and can help reduce the risk of cancer.

Leftovers tip Try these tuna patties on a nice crusty bun for lunch or freeze them in resealable plastic bags for a later meal.

Three 5-ounce cans tuna packed
    in water, drained
1 green onion, finely chopped
½ teaspoon minced garlic
3 eggs, beaten

Juice of ½ large lemon
1 tablespoon chopped fresh parsley
1 teaspoon chopped fresh dill
Nonstick cooking spray

1. In a large bowl, combine all the ingredients except the cooking spray.
2. Form the mixture into 12 equal patties, each about 2 inches in diameter.
3. Place the patties on a plate, cover, and chill in the refrigerator until firm, about 1 hour.
4. In a large skillet over medium-high heat, add a light coat of cooking spray and cook the tuna patties, turning once, until lightly browned, about 4 minutes per side.
5. Serve 3 tuna cakes per portion.

Serves 4. Prep time 15 minutes. Cook time 8 minutes.

Calories **200** / Calories from fat **43** / Total fat **4.8g** / Saturated fat **1.4g** / Trans fat **0.0g** / Sodium **116mg** / Carbs **1.0g** / Sugars **0.0g** / Protein **36.5g**

Shrimp with Roasted Tomatoes and Feta Cheese

Shrimp is a low-fat and low-calorie seafood. It is very high in selenium, vitamin B_{12}, protein, and phosphorus, as well as antioxidants that are usually associated with produce. This popular crustacean can cut the risk of cancer, heart disease, and type 2 diabetes. Try to buy wild-caught shrimp to avoid issues sometimes found in farmed shrimp, such as parasites and virus contamination.

Nutrition tip If you are on a low-cholesterol diet, shrimp may not be the best choice for you. A four-ounce portion of shrimp contains 220 milligrams of cholesterol.

6 large tomatoes, cut into eighths

3 teaspoons olive oil

3 teaspoons minced garlic

Freshly ground black pepper

42 medium shrimp, peeled and deveined

½ cup chopped fresh parsley

4 teaspoons lemon juice

½ cup crumbled low-sodium feta cheese

1. Preheat the oven to 450°F.
2. In a large bowl, toss the tomatoes with the oil and garlic until well coated.
3. Transfer the tomatoes to a 9-by-13-inch glass baking dish and season with pepper to taste.
4. Bake the tomatoes in the oven for 20 minutes.
5. Add the shrimp, parsley, and lemon juice to the tomatoes and stir to combine, then sprinkle the feta over the top.
6. Return the dish to the oven and bake until the shrimp are cooked through, about 15 minutes. Serve hot.

Serves 6. Prep time 15 minutes. Cook time 35 minutes.

Calories **374** / Calories from fat **91** / Total fat **10.1g** / Saturated fat **3.1g** / Trans fat **0.0g** / Sodium **793mg** / Carbs **11.3g** / Sugars **7.3g** / Protein **58.9g**

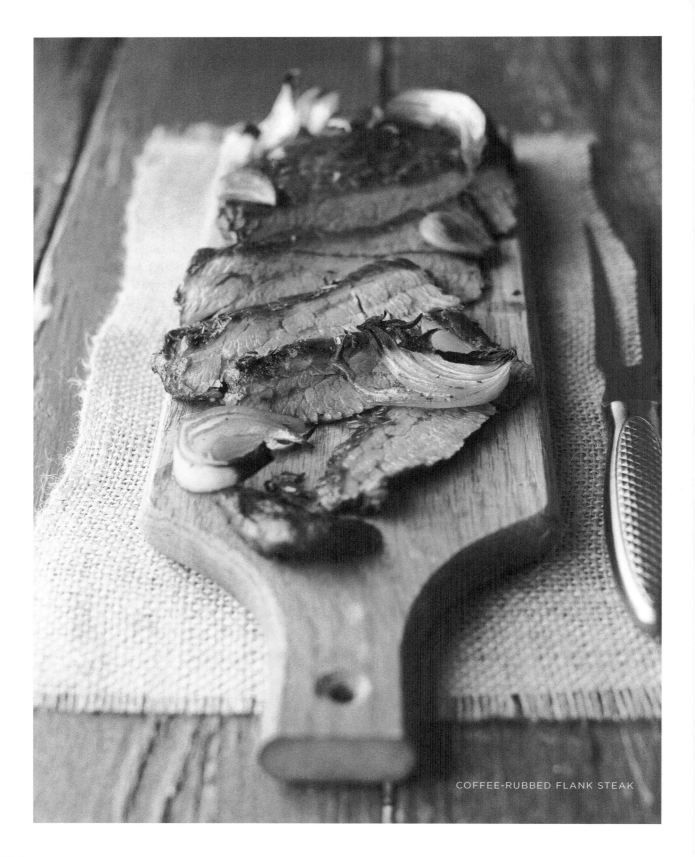

COFFEE-RUBBED FLANK STEAK

CHAPTER TWELVE

Meat and Poultry

Chicken Ratatouille

Gluten-free
Low-sodium

MEAT AND
POULTRY

Zucchini is a vegetable that people either love or hate. It is often the texture that gets the thumbs down, because it can be unpleasantly soft and spongy if the vegetable is too ripe. Although winter squashes seem starchier than summer squashes, both get about 85 percent of their calories from carbohydrates. Summer squash (zucchini and yellow summer squash) is an excellent source of manganese, copper, magnesium, and vitamins A and C, as well as fiber.

Shopping tip When choosing your zucchini, look for vegetables that seem heavy for their size and have an unmarked, shiny skin. Do not purchase larger zucchini thinking you will need less of them, because the big ones are usually fibrous and have tough seeds.

1 teaspoon olive oil

Two 6-ounce boneless, skinless chicken
  breasts, diced

1 small sweet onion, peeled and sliced

2 teaspoons minced garlic

2 zucchini, unpeeled, sliced lengthwise,
  then cut into half moons

1 small eggplant, diced

2 red bell peppers, seeded and diced

4 large tomatoes, chopped

2 tablespoons chopped fresh basil

1 tablespoon chopped fresh thyme

Pinch of crushed red pepper flakes

1. In a large skillet over medium heat, heat the oil and sauté the chicken breast pieces until browned and cooked through, about 5 minutes.
2. Add the onion and garlic and sauté until softened, about 3 minutes.
3. Stir in the zucchini, eggplant, and bell peppers, and cook for 15 minutes, stirring occasionally.
4. Stir in the tomatoes, basil, thyme, and red pepper flakes, combining well, and cook for 5 more minutes.
5. Serve the ratatouille plain or over rice.

Serves 6. Prep time 15 minutes. Cook time 30 minutes.

Calories **285** / Calories from fat **75** / Total fat **8.4g** / Saturated fat **2.0g** / Sodium **93mg** / Carbs **13.2g** / Sugars **13.2g** / Protein **30.3g**

Jerk Chicken

This style of seasoning is Jamaican and was developed to preserve meat with spices, salt, and peppers. This recipe does not use as much salt as some, but the flavoring is pungent. Chilies and allspice are traditional ingredients in jerk marinades. Be careful, because habañeros are very hot. You can adjust the heat by using milder or hotter chilies depending on your preference.

Shopping tip Turbinado is a less processed variety of cane sugar. It is brown and comes in large crystals—the color comes from its molasses content. It's turning up in more and more supermarkets, sometimes packaged as "sugar in the raw."

Four 5-ounce boneless, skinless
    chicken breasts
1 small sweet onion, peeled and cut
    into chunks
3 habañero peppers, halved lengthwise
    and seeded
3 teaspoons minced garlic
3 tablespoons fresh lime juice

1 tablespoon olive oil, plus more to
    oil the grill
1 tablespoon turbinado sugar
1 tablespoon chopped fresh thyme
1 tablespoon ground allspice
1 teaspoon freshly ground black pepper
½ teaspoon ground nutmeg
½ teaspoon ground cinnamon

1. Put two chicken breasts each in two large, zipper-top plastic bags and set them aside.
2. In a food processor, combine all the remaining ingredients and pulse until the marinade is very well blended, about 1 minute.
3. Divide the jerk marinade evenly between the two bags of chicken, squeeze as much air as possible out of the bags, and seal them. Squeeze and shake the bags to distribute the marinade evenly on the surface of the chicken breasts.
4. Put the bags in the refrigerator for at least 4 hours or overnight.
5. Preheat a barbecue to medium-high heat and brush the grill lightly with olive oil. Or preheat your oven to 400°F and grease a heavy, ovenproof skillet with olive oil.

continued ➤

6. Take the chicken out of the refrigerator about 15 minutes before cooking and then remove the chicken from the bags.
7. On the barbecue, grill the chicken, turning at least once, until cooked through, about 6 minutes per side. Or on the stovetop, heat the greased ovenproof skillet over medium-high heat and brown the chicken in the skillet, turning once, about 4 minutes per side. Then put the skillet in the oven and roast until the chicken is cooked though, about 10 minutes. Let the chicken rest for about 5 minutes before serving.

Serves 4. Prep time 30 minutes, plus marinating time. Cook time 20 minutes.

Calories **374** / Calories from fat **160** / Total fat **17.8g** / Saturated fat **4.0g** / Trans fat **0.0g** / Sodium **132mg** / Carbs **9.0g** / Sugars **1.4g** / Protein **41.6g**

Greek Chicken Breasts

Stuffed chicken breasts look like they are incredibly hard to make, but this simple recipe takes only about 15 minutes to put together. The Kalamata olives give this dish a nice briny flavor, and they are also a good source of fiber, iron, and vitamin E. Olives are heart-friendly, promote good digestion, and boost the immune system.

Shopping tip When selecting olives, make sure they are firm with no softness or mushiness. Olives purchased in jars can be kept in the refrigerator for several months, but those bought from open olive bars in the supermarket will only keep for about two weeks. Make sure there is enough brine or liquid in your storage container to cover the olives.

1 large red bell pepper

1 teaspoon olive oil, plus more for the grill

4 tablespoons crumbled low-sodium feta cheese

3 Kalamata olives, pitted and finely chopped

2 tablespoons chopped fresh basil

Pinch of freshly ground black pepper

Four 5-ounce skinless, boneless chicken breasts

1. Preheat the oven to 400°F. Lightly coat the red pepper in 1 teaspoon of olive oil.
2. In a small baking dish, roast the red pepper in the oven until tender, about 30 minutes.
3. Remove the pepper from the oven and transfer it to a small bowl. Cover the bowl tightly with plastic wrap and set aside for about 10 minutes to loosen the pepper's skin.
4. Peel and seed the pepper using your fingers, then dice it.
5. In a small bowl, combine the roasted pepper, feta, olives, basil, and pepper until well mixed.
6. Chill the filling in the refrigerator for about 10 minutes.
7. Preheat a barbecue to medium-high heat and brush the grill rack with olive oil. Or place a large, heavy skillet over medium-high heat on the stove and lightly oil the skillet with olive oil.

continued ➤

Greek Chicken Breasts *continued*

8. Cut a slit horizontally in each chicken breast, creating a pocket in the middle.
9. Spoon about 2 tablespoons of the filling into each breast pocket and secure the opening with a wooden toothpick.
10. On the barbecue, grill the chicken until completely cooked through, about 10 minutes per side. Or on the stovetop, place the chicken breasts in the skillet and pan fry the breasts until cooked through, turning once, about 10 minutes per side.
11. Remove the chicken from the heat and let stand for 10 minutes.
12. Remove the toothpicks and serve.

Serves 4. Prep time 15 minutes. Cook time 50 minutes.

Calories **188** / Calories from fat **58** / Total fat **6.4g** / Saturated fat **2.6g** / Trans fat **0.0g** / Sodium **184mg** / Carbs **2.7g** / Sugar **0.0g** / Protein **33.5g**

Chicken Florentine

When you see the word "Florentine" in a recipe, it usually means that spinach is a key ingredient. Spinach is a super food, meaning it is packed with healthy nutrients and antioxidants. Spinach is rich in beta-carotene, protein, lutein, calcium, folic acid, potassium, iron, and vitamins A, C, and E.

Nutrition tip Spinach can promote overall healing as well as specifically reduce the pain associated with arthritis and the risk of high blood pressure and cancer. Spinach is also an efficient liver cleanser.

1 teaspoon olive oil

Four 4-ounce boneless, skinless
    chicken breasts

3 large tomatoes, finely chopped

1 tablespoon chopped fresh basil

1 tablespoon chopped fresh oregano

1 teaspoon minced garlic

2 cups packed baby spinach

4 teaspoons grated Parmesan cheese

1. In a large skillet over medium-high heat, heat the olive oil and brown the chicken breasts in the skillet, about 6 minutes per side. Add the tomatoes, basil, oregano, and garlic, and reduce the heat to medium.
2. Cover the skillet and cook the chicken for about 15 minutes.
3. Add the spinach and cover the skillet again. Cook for 5 more minutes or until the spinach is wilted.
4. Top with Parmesan cheese and serve.

Serves 4. Prep time 10 minutes. Cook time 30 minutes.

Calories **336** / Calories from fat **142** / Total fat **15.8g** / Saturated fat **5.5g** / Trans fat **0.0g** / Sodium **415mg** / Carbs **4.0g** / Sugars **1.6g** / Protein **43.2g**

Turkey with Apricot Chutney

The easiest description of chutney is that it is a spicy cooked salsa that can be savory, but is usually more on the sweet side. Apricots are a great ingredient for a chutney because they have a firm texture that does not break down completely, and a hint of natural acid to cut the sweetness. Apricots are a lovely rosy gold color, which means they are high in antioxidants—the deeper the color, the greater the concentration of antioxidants. Apricots have powerful cancer-fighting properties due to their high lycopene content.

Leftovers tip If you have chutney left over after your meal, try it as a spread on sandwiches, a dipping sauce, or as a glaze on roasted pork or chicken. Store the chutney in the refrigerator in a sealed container for up to a week.

6 ripe apricots, pitted and diced

¼ cup unsweetened apple juice

¼ small sweet onion, finely chopped

2 tablespoons honey

1 tablespoon grated fresh ginger

1 tablespoon chopped fresh thyme

1 tablespoon balsamic vinegar

1 teaspoon freshly grated lemon zest

Juice of 1 lime

1 pound whole boneless turkey breast, skin removed, trimmed of visible fat

1 teaspoon smoked paprika

½ teaspoon ground cumin

1 teaspoon olive oil

1. In a small saucepan, combine the apricots, apple juice, onion, honey, ginger, thyme, vinegar, lemon zest, and lime juice.
2. Cook over medium heat, stirring constantly until the apricots become soft and mushy, about 10 minutes.
3. Remove the chutney from the heat and set aside.
4. Preheat the oven to 375°F.
5. Season the turkey breast with the paprika and cumin.
6. In a large ovenproof skillet over medium-high heat, heat the oil and pan sear the turkey on all sides, about 5 minutes per side.

7. Put the skillet in the oven and roast the turkey until the breast is cooked through and the internal temperature reaches 165°F, about 45 minutes.
8. Let the turkey breast rest for about 10 minutes before carving it into slices.
9. Serve with the chutney.

Serves 4. Prep time 15 minutes. Cook time 1 hour and 5 minutes.

Calories **204** / Calories from fat **32** / Total fat **3.5g** / Saturated fat **0.6g** / Trans fat **0.0g** / Sodium **1154mg** / Carbs **24.2g** / Sugars **19.5g** / Protein **20.5g**

Pork Tenderloin with Squash Salsa

Pork is a very healthy clean eating choice, but is often forgotten in favor of chicken and fish. Pork is a red meat, but it does not have the same nutritional profile as beef. Pork tenderloin is actually as lean as a skinless chicken breast and has fewer calories. Lean cuts of pork, such as chops and tenderloins, also have less total fat and calories than lean beef.

Cooking tip The days of cooking pork until it was dry and an unappetizing gray are gone, because trichinosis is no longer a risk. Pork can actually be served with a hint of pink in the middle, especially if the cut is thick, such as a pork tenderloin.

½ small butternut squash, peeled and
    diced into ¼-inch cubes
2 tablespoons olive oil, divided
1 apple, peeled, cored, and diced
1 small red bell pepper, seeded
    and finely chopped
1 green onion, finely chopped

1 tablespoon fresh lime juice
1 teaspoon chopped fresh thyme
1 teaspoon honey
½ teaspoon nutmeg
Freshly ground black pepper
Two 10-ounce pork tenderloins,
    trimmed of fat

1. Preheat the oven to 400°F. Line a baking sheet with foil and set it aside.
2. In a small bowl, toss the squash with 1 tablespoon of the olive oil.
3. Transfer the squash to the prepared baking sheet and bake until cooked but not mushy, about 20 minutes.
4. Transfer the squash to a large bowl and let it cool for about 15 minutes.
5. Add the apple, bell pepper, onion, lime juice, thyme, honey, and nutmeg to the squash and stir to combine well. Season the salsa with black pepper to taste.
6. Store the salsa in the refrigerator until you are ready to serve the pork.
7. In a large skillet over medium-high heat, heat the remaining tablespoon of oil.

8. Season the pork lightly with pepper and pan fry the meat, turning to brown each side, until it is cooked through and the internal temperature is 160°F, about 20 minutes total.
9. Let the pork rest for about 10 minutes before cutting each one in half.
10. Transfer each half to an individual plate and top with salsa. Serve immediately.

Serves 4. Prep time 15 minutes. Cook time 40 minutes.

Calories **417** / Calories from fat **169** / Total fat **18.8g** / Saturated fat **5.2g** / Trans fat **0.0g** / Sodium **96mg** / Carbs **17.6g** / Sugars **8.9g** / Protein **43.4g**

MEAT AND POULTRY

Marinated Pork Chops with Grilled Peaches

The marinade for these thick chops is the perfect blend of sweetness and acid. Many marinades use acids to break the protein bonds in the meat, creating a tender finished product. You have to be careful not to marinate meats such as chicken and pork in an acidic marinade for too long, because time can cause the bonds to tighten up again and your meat will be dry and tough.

Cooking tip Reserve about 3 tablespoons of the marinade before adding the pork chops to the bag, and brush the extra marinade on the peaches before grilling them.

¼ cup balsamic vinegar

¼ cup olive oil, plus more for the grill

2 tablespoons honey

1 tablespoon chopped fresh thyme, divided

½ teaspoon chopped fresh rosemary, divided

Four 5-ounce boneless pork chops, trimmed of visible fat

2 ripe peaches, halved and pitted

Freshly ground black pepper

1. In a large zipper-top plastic bag, combine the vinegar, olive oil, honey, half of the thyme, and half of the rosemary, and shake to blend.
2. Add the pork chops to the vinegar mixture and squeeze the bag to coat all the sides of the meat with marinade.
3. Squeeze as much air out of the bag as possible, seal it, and place the bag in the refrigerator to marinate for at least 1 hour and no more than 4 hours.
4. Preheat a barbecue to medium-high heat and brush the grill lightly with olive oil. Or preheat the broiler and lightly oil a broiler pan.
5. On the barbecue, grill the peaches cut-side down until very tender. Or in the oven, broil them for 2 minutes per side.
6. Remove the peaches from the heat to a medium bowl and set aside to cool for 5 minutes.

7. Chop the peaches and add the remaining thyme and rosemary. Season with pepper to taste and set aside. Take the pork chops out of the bag and shake off any excess marinade.

8. On the barbecue, grill the pork until cooked through but still juicy (160°F on a meat thermometer), about 5 minutes per side. Or in the oven, broil the pork until it is cooked through, about 6 minutes per side.

9. Remove the chops from the heat and let them sit for 5 minutes.

10. Serve topped with the grilled peaches.

Serves 4. Prep time 10 minutes, plus marinating time. Cook time 15 minutes.

Calories **367** / Calories from fat **160** / Total fat **17.8g** / Saturated fat **3.5g** / Trans fat **0.1g** / Sodium **82mg** / Carbs **14.0g** / Sugars **12.8g** / Protein **37.7g**

Sweet Pepper Sauté with Sirloin

Sweet bell peppers are the supporting ingredient of the lean sirloin, but they more than hold their own with respect to nutrition. This recipe features every color of pepper except green, and each color has different phytonutrients. All the sweet bell peppers are high in potassium, zinc, calcium, magnesium, and vitamins A, B, C, and E. They can help boost the immune system, prevent cataracts, and reduce the risk of heart disease, blood clots, and cancer.

Leftovers tip The pepper sauté makes a delicious, healthy pasta sauce, especially if you add a bit of blue cheese to the finished dish.

1 pound boneless top sirloin steak, about 1 inch thick, trimmed of visible fat

1 tablespoon olive oil, plus more for brushing the steak

Salt and freshly ground black pepper

1 small red onion, peeled and thinly sliced

2 teaspoons minced garlic

2 yellow bell peppers, seeded and thinly sliced

2 red bell peppers, seeded and thinly sliced

1 orange bell pepper, seeded and thinly sliced

1 cup baby spinach

1 cup halved cherry tomatoes

½ cup crumbled blue cheese

1. Preheat a barbecue to medium-high heat or preheat the broiler.
2. Lightly brush the steak on both sides with the olive oil and season with salt and pepper to taste.
3. On the barbecue, grill the steak, turning once, until it reaches the desired doneness, about 5 minutes per side for medium (160°F). Or in the oven, broil the steak, turning once, until it reaches the desired doneness. For medium, broil the meat 6 minutes per side or until a meat thermometer reads 160°F.
4. Transfer the steak to a cutting board and let it rest for at least 10 minutes before slicing it against the grain into 16 slices.

5. In a large skillet on the stove over medium heat, heat the remaining tablespoon of oil and sauté the onion and garlic until softened, 3 minutes.
6. Add the peppers and sauté until they are tender but still crisp, about 5 minutes.
7. Add the spinach and cherry tomatoes and stir until the spinach is wilted, about 2 minutes.
8. Season the mixture with pepper to taste.
9. Divide the sautéed peppers among 4 plates and top with about 4 steak pieces each and a sprinkle of blue cheese.

Serves 4. Prep time 15 minutes. Cook time 20 minutes.

Calories **364** / Calories from fat **144** / Total fat **16.0g** / Saturated fat **6.4g** / Sodium **324mg** / Carbs **13.2g** / Sugars **8.1g** / Protein **40.2g**

Coffee-Rubbed Flank Steak

If you are a meat-eater, you might be surprised to discover that coffee is a great marinade for steaks. It imparts a lovely smoky taste to the meat without any chemicals or preservatives. This recipe uses ground coffee beans as a base; if you like the taste of the coffee-accented meat, you could also try soaking your beef in brewed coffee. Make sure you don't use hot coffee for your marinade or you will cook the meat.

Shopping tip Flank steak is an ideal, inexpensive grilling choice if you are marinating your meat. Keep in mind that the tougher cuts of meat, like flank steak, are also more flavorful than the tender cuts, like tenderloin.

3 teaspoons minced garlic

¼ cup whole espresso coffee beans

2 tablespoons chopped fresh parsley

2 tablespoons chopped fresh rosemary

2 teaspoons freshly ground black pepper

3 tablespoons balsamic vinegar

2 tablespoons turbinado sugar

1 tablespoon olive oil, plus more
   for the grill

1 pound flank steak, trimmed of visible fat

1. In a food processor, combine the garlic, espresso beans, parsley, and rosemary and pulse until the beans are coarsely ground.
2. Add the pepper, vinegar, sugar, and olive oil and pulse until the marinade is well blended.
3. Pour the coffee marinade into a large zipper-top plastic bag, add the flank steak, and squeeze the excess air out of the bag and seal it.
4. Marinate the steak in the refrigerator for at least 4 hours or overnight, turning the bag occasionally.
5. Preheat a barbecue to medium-high heat and brush the grill with olive oil. Or preheat the broiler and brush a broiler pan with olive oil.
6. Remove the steak from the bag and shake off the excess marinade.
7. On the barbecue, grill the steak, turning once, until it reaches the desired doneness, about 5 minutes per side for medium (160°F). Or in the oven, broil the steak, turning once, until it is the desired doneness, about 6 minutes per side.

8. Transfer the steak to a cutting board and let the meat rest for at least 10 minutes before slicing it against the grain.
9. Serve the steak with a mixed green salad or your favorite side dish.

Serves 4. Prep time 20 minutes, plus marinating time. Cook time 10 minutes.

Calories **312** / Calories from fat **151** / Total fat **16.7g** / Saturated fat **5.0g** / Trans fat **0.0g** /
Sodium **68mg** / Carbs **7.1g** / Sugars **4.5g** / Protein **31.9g**

Beef Tenderloin with Onion Marmalade

This marmalade is outrageously flavorful, and it has a surprisingly sweet taste that pairs well with the tenderloin. The trick to a perfectly balanced and delicious onion marmalade is slow cooking the onions until all the natural sugars are released, so don't rush the process. You can use any onion in this recipe rather than the red ones—such as the fancy Vidalia or the plain yellow ones—but the color will be lighter.

Cooking tip You can leave out the honey entirely if your marmalade is already sweet and rich after caramelizing.

1 teaspoon olive oil, plus more for the grill

2 large red onions, peeled and diced

2 tablespoons unsweetened apple juice

3 teaspoons red wine vinegar

2 tablespoons honey

1 tablespoon chopped fresh thyme

Pinch of salt

Pinch of freshly ground black pepper

Four 4-ounce beef tenderloin steaks, each about 1 inch thick and trimmed of fat

1. In a large saucepan over medium-low heat, heat the oil and sauté the red onion until it is very soft and lightly caramelized, about 1 hour, stirring frequently.
2. Add the juice, vinegar, honey, thyme, salt, and pepper.
3. Reduce the heat to low and continue to cook, stirring frequently, until most of the liquid evaporates and the marmalade is sticky and thick, about 10 minutes. Remove the pan from the heat and set it aside.
4. Preheat a barbecue to medium-high heat and brush the grill with olive oil. Or preheat the broiler and lightly oil a broiling pan.
5. On the barbecue, grill the tenderloin, turning once, until it is the desired doneness, about 5 minutes per side for medium (160°F). Or in the oven, broil the tenderloin until is it the desired doneness, turning once, about 6 minutes per side.

6. Transfer the tenderloin to a cutting board and let it rest for at least 10 minutes.
7. Serve topped with the onion marmalade.

Serves 4. Prep time 30 minutes. Cook time 1 hour and 20 minutes.

Calories **291** / Calories from fat **75** / Total fat **8.3g** / Saturated fat **2.9g** / Trans fat **0.0g** / Sodium **223mg** / Carbs **17.1g** / Sugars **12.7g** / Protein **35.0g**

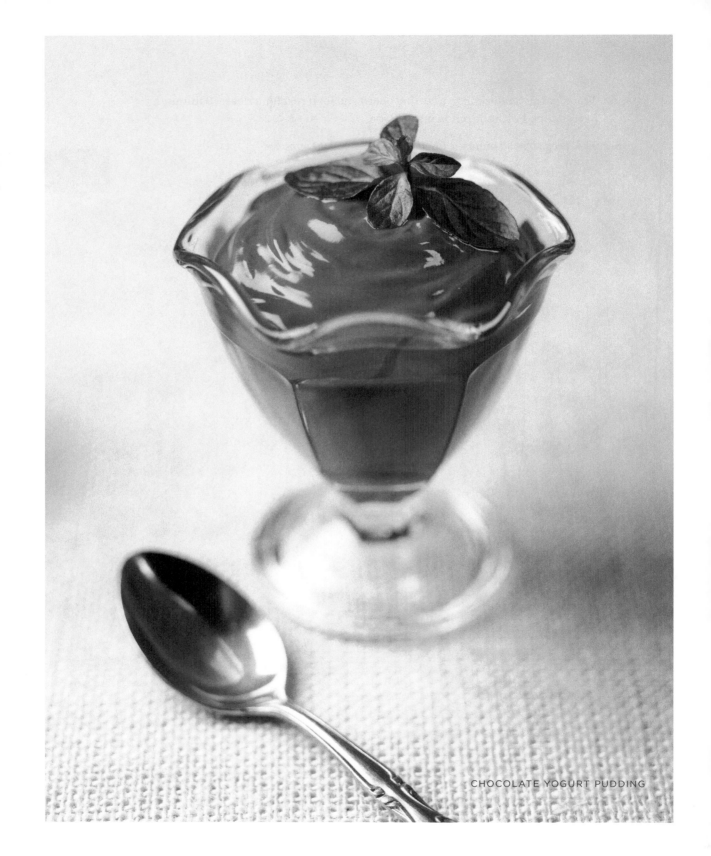

CHOCOLATE YOGURT PUDDING

CHAPTER THIRTEEN

Desserts

Citrus Coconut Mousse

This dessert is like an infusion of the tropics, with lemon, orange, and coconut. Coconut is a high-calorie and high-fat addition to the recipe, but it is also packed with fiber and contains no trans fats. Shredded coconut can help improve digestion, and it is a delicious energy booster.

Diet tip This dish is not appropriate for a vegetarian or vegan diet because it contains gelatin, which is an animal-based product. But there are vegan gelling agents: agar-agar and carrageen are both derived from seaweed. Many kosher gelatins use these products, and are vegan.

3 teaspoons fresh lemon juice

1 teaspoon fresh orange juice

1 teaspoon unflavored gelatin

1 cup unsweetened almond milk

3 tablespoons turbinado sugar

½ teaspoon pure vanilla extract

3 pasteurized egg whites

1 small mango, peeled, pitted, and diced

¼ cup unsweetened shredded coconut

1. In a small bowl, mix the lemon and orange juices and then sprinkle the gelatin over them. Let the mixture stand for 5 minutes.
2. In a small saucepan over medium heat, heat the almond milk.
3. When the milk starts to bubble around the sides of the pan, add the sugar and vanilla extract and stir until the sugar is completely dissolved.
4. Remove the mixture from the heat and whisk in the gelatin mixture.
5. Transfer the almond milk mixture to a large bowl and chill in the refrigerator for about 15 minutes.
6. In a medium bowl, beat the egg whites with an electric beater or whisk until soft peaks form.
7. Remove the almond milk mixture from the refrigerator and fold in the beaten egg whites in three increments, keeping as much volume as possible.

8. Divide the mousse among four serving dishes and place them in the refrigerator to set for at least 2 hours or overnight.
9. Serve with the mango and coconut.

Serves 4. Prep time 30 minutes, plus setting time. Cook time 10 minutes.

Calories **100** / Calories from fat **17** / Total fat **1.9g** / Saturated fat **1.5g** / Sodium **49mg** / Carbs **14.8g** / Sugars **15.1g** / Protein **4.7g**

Chocolate Yogurt Pudding

This decadent pudding tastes a little like a rich chocolate cheesecake and is much simpler to make. Be sure to use dark chocolate, at least 70 percent cocoa, for this dessert because it is very healthy in small amounts. Dark chocolate is much lower in fat and sugar than milk chocolate, and may lower cholesterol levels, reduce the risk of heart disease, and prevent cognitive decline. Serve this pudding topped with antioxidant-rich berries for a super healthy dessert.

Shopping tip Choose the highest quality chocolate possible for this dessert because the taste and texture will be superior. If you can find it, try single-plantation chocolate because the taste of chocolate can be affected by where the beans come from, similar to wine and grapes.

2 cups vanilla Greek yogurt

4 ounces dark chocolate,
    coarsely chopped

½ teaspoon pure vanilla extract

1. Line a medium fine-mesh sieve with cheesecloth.
2. Place the sieve over a bowl and spoon the yogurt into the cheesecloth.
3. Put the bowl and sieve in the refrigerator for about 1 hour to drain.
4. Transfer the drained yogurt to a medium bowl and whisk the yogurt for about 30 seconds.
5. Let the yogurt sit on the counter for about 15 minutes to come to room temperature.
6. Place the chocolate in a small heatproof bowl and melt it in the microwave or over a pan of simmering water.
7. Whisk the melted chocolate and vanilla into the yogurt until very well blended.
8. Spoon the chocolate pudding into 4 serving bowls, cover them, and put them in the refrigerator until you are ready to serve them. They will keep overnight.

Serves 4. Prep time 15 minutes. Cook time 5 minutes.

Calories **271** / Calories from fat **94** / Total fat **11.4g** / Saturated fat **7.1g** / Trans fat **0.0g** / Sodium **73mg** / Carbs **33.5g** / Sugars **30.7g** / Protein **11.2g**

Simple Banana Strawberry Ice Cream

Gluten-free
Low-fat
Low-sodium
Nightshade-free
Vegan
Vegetarian

DESSERTS

You do not need an ice cream maker to create this creamy cold dessert—just a blender. Bananas are a very good source of potassium, fiber, manganese, and vitamins B_6 and C. They also contain tryptophan, which can improve your mood. Bananas help improve digestion and protect against cardiovascular disease, type 2 diabetes, and cancer.

Cooking tip For best results, take the frozen bananas out of the freezer and let them sit at room temperature for about 30 minutes, until they are soft enough to blend into a creamy dessert.

2 frozen bananas, peeled before freezing
½ cup frozen strawberries, cut in half
    before freezing

1 teaspoon pure vanilla extract

1. In a food processor, combine the bananas and strawberries and pulse until smooth and creamy, about 2 minutes.
2. Add the vanilla and pulse until well combined.
3. Serve immediately or store the ice cream in the freezer in a sealed container for up to 1 week.

Serves 4. Prep time 15 minutes.

Calories **62** / Calories from fat **2** / Total fat **0.2g** / Trans fat **0.0g** / Sodium **1mg** / Carbs **15.3g** / Sugars **8.5g** / Protein **0.7g**

Strawberry Crisp

Strawberries are very high in ellagic acid, vitamin C, beta-carotene, iron, folic acid, and potassium. They can boost the immune system, help stabilize blood sugar, and cut the risk of heart disease, cognitive decline, and some types of cancer. They are truly a nutritional powerhouse.

Shopping tip Strawberries have a very short shelf life and can start losing vitamin C after sitting in your refrigerator for two days. Try to find local organic berries in the early summer for the best taste and quality.

Nonstick cooking spray
½ cup rolled oats
¼ cup unsweetened shredded coconut
¼ cup finely chopped raw pecans
¼ cup turbinado sugar, divided
¼ teaspoon ground cinnamon

¼ teaspoon ground nutmeg
2 tablespoons pure maple syrup
1 tablespoon coconut oil, melted
4 cups sliced strawberries
1 tablespoon fresh lemon juice
1 tablespoon arrowroot powder

1. Preheat the oven to 350°F. Lightly coat a 9-by-13-inch glass baking dish with cooking spray and set aside.
2. In a medium bowl, mix together the oats, coconut, pecans, half of the turbinado sugar, cinnamon, and nutmeg until well mixed.
3. Stir in the maple syrup and coconut oil and toss together until the mixture resembles coarse crumbs.
4. In a large bowl, toss together the strawberries, lemon juice, remaining sugar, and arrowroot until well mixed.
5. Spoon the strawberry mixture into the baking dish and top evenly with the oat mixture.
6. Bake for 15 minutes.
7. Serve warm.

Serves 6. Prep time 20 minutes. Cook time 15 minutes.

Calories **274** / Calories from fat **126** / Total fat **14.0g** / Saturated fat **7.6g** / Trans fat **0.0g** / Sodium **6mg** / Carbs **24.5g** / Sugars **14.0g** / Protein **3.6g**

Pumpkin Pie Mousse

Pumpkin and warm spices are a traditional combination found in pies, cakes, and breads. This mousse is a little like pumpkin pie without the crust, and is a great deal healthier. Pumpkin is often thought of as a vegetable, but it is actually a fruit. Pumpkin is a wonderful source of beta-carotene, vitamins B, C, D, and E, and iron, potassium, and copper. It can cut the risk of developing quite a few diseases, including strokes, kidney stones, cancer, heart disease, and insomnia.

Cooking tip Silken tofu is a fabulous, fat-free way to create creamy, thick desserts that have the lightness associated with whipped cream and beaten egg whites.

One 15-ounce can plain pumpkin purée
One 10½-ounce package silken tofu,
    well drained
⅓ cup pure maple syrup
1 teaspoon ground cinnamon

¼ teaspoon ground nutmeg
¼ teaspoon ground ginger
Pinch of ground cloves
¼ cup plain Greek yogurt

1. In a food processor, combine the pumpkin and tofu and pulse until smooth, about 30 seconds.
2. Add the remaining ingredients except the yogurt and pulse until very smooth, about 30 seconds.
3. Put the mousse in the refrigerator in a sealed container for at least 4 hours.
4. Drain any liquid from the top of the mousse and spoon the mousse into serving dishes.
5. Top with a little Greek yogurt and serve.

Serves 5. Prep time 10 minutes, plus setting time.

Calories **97** / Calories from fat **11** / Total fat **2.1g** / Saturated fat **0.7g** / Trans fat **0.0g** / Sodium **10mg** / Carbs **24.8g** / Sugars **16.5g** / Protein **4.7g**

Pecan Fruit Salad

What is a perfect clean eating dessert? Fruit salad, of course! Fresh, delicious fruit is a sweet end to a meal, and this version adds a tiny surprise crunch of spicy caramelized nuts to enhance the flavor and texture. You can use any fruit for this dish, depending on your own personal preference, but try to get a nice assortment of colors for visual impact.

Leftovers tip Store any remaining fruit salad in the refrigerator in a sealed container. It will make for a great breakfast the next morning and an energy-packed start to the day.

1 cup halved strawberries

1 kiwi, peeled and sliced

1 peach, pitted and diced

1 cup raspberries

1 mango, peeled, pitted, and diced

1 teaspoon honey

¼ teaspoon cayenne pepper

¼ cup chopped pecans

1. Preheat the oven to broil.
2. In a large bowl, toss the strawberries, kiwi, peach, raspberries, and mango together, and set aside.
3. In a small bowl, stir together the honey and cayenne pepper.
4. Add the pecans to the honey mixture and stir to coat.
5. On a small baking sheet, spread the nuts and broil until they are toasted and lightly caramelized, about 1 minute.
6. Stir the toasted nuts into the fruit salad and serve.

Serves 4. Prep time 15 minutes. Cook time 1 minute.

Calories **137** / Calories from fat **49** / Total fat **5.5g** / Saturated fat **0.0g** / Trans fats **0.0g** / Sodium **2mg** / Carbs **22.8g** / Sugars **16.4g** / Protein **1.9g**

Oatmeal Maple Cookies

Desserts don't have to be fancy or elaborate to be successful. Sometimes a simple, rich cookie served with an herbal tea is the best end to a good meal. These cookies will remind you of your grandmother's recipe because they have a melt-in-your-mouth texture and a hint of maple sweetness. If you are watching your fat consumption, you can omit the coconut oil in the ingredients and double the applesauce, but this will change the texture a little.

Diet tip If you want a gluten-free cookie, substitute almond flour for the whole-wheat flour, and make sure your oats are gluten-free as well.

3 cups rolled oats

1½ cups whole-wheat flour

1 teaspoon ground cinnamon

½ teaspoon baking soda

Pinch of sea salt

½ cup pure maple syrup

½ cup unsweetened applesauce

¼ cup coconut oil

1 teaspoon pure vanilla extract

1 large banana, mashed

1. Preheat the oven to 375°F. Line a baking sheet with foil or parchment paper and set it aside.
2. In a large bowl, stir together the oats, flour, cinnamon, baking soda, and salt.
3. In a medium bowl, stir together the remaining ingredients until there are no banana lumps.
4. Add the wet ingredients to the dry ingredients and stir to combine well.
5. Drop the batter by tablespoons onto the baking sheet, about 12 per batch.
6. Bake the cookies until golden brown, about 10 minutes.
7. Repeat with the remaining batter.
8. Store the cookies in a sealed container for up to 1 week.

Makes 24 cookies. Prep time 10 minutes. Cook time 20 minutes.

Calories **112** / Calories from fat **27** / Total fat **3.1g** / Saturated fat **2.1g** / Trans fat **0.0g** / Sodium **41mg** / Carbs **19.3g** / Sugars **5.2g** / Protein **2.2g**

Low-fat
Low-sodium
Nightshade-free
Vegan
Vegetarian

DESSERTS

Rhubarb Apple Brown Betty

Rhubarb looks a little like reddish green celery, but it is cooked more like a fruit in pies, stews, and cakes. Rhubarb can be incredibly tart. This recipe mellows the flavor with the addition of sweet apple and apple juice. If you want the fruit layer of this crisp to be less tart, add a couple tablespoons of maple syrup to the stewed mixture. Rhubarb is very low in calories and is a great source of lutein, calcium, and vitamin K.

Shopping tip Buy your rhubarb from late spring to late summer and always remove the leaves because they contain oxalic acid, which can be toxic.

For the filling:
4 cups diced rhubarb
2 large apples, peeled, cored, and diced
½ cup unsweetened apple juice
1 teaspoon ground cinnamon
½ teaspoon ground nutmeg
1 tablespoon cornstarch

For the topping:
¾ cup rolled oats
¼ cup chopped pecans
½ cup uncooked quinoa, rinsed
4 dates, chopped

To make the filling:
1. In a large saucepan over medium heat, combine all the filling ingredients and bring to a boil.
2. Reduce the heat to low and simmer the mixture, stirring frequently, for about 1 hour, until the filling is thick and stewed.

To make the brown betty:
1. While the rhubarb filling is stewing, in a food processor combine all the topping ingredients and pulse until it resembles coarse crumbs. Set aside.
2. Preheat the oven to 350°F.
3. When the filling is cooked, pour it into a 9-by-13-inch glass baking dish and sprinkle the topping over the filling.
4. Bake the brown betty until golden and bubbly, about 20 minutes.

5. Remove the dessert from the oven, and let it cool on a wire rack for about 30 minutes, and serve warm or cool.
6. Store any leftovers in a sealed container in the refrigerator for up to 5 days.

Serves 6. Prep time 15 minutes. Cook time 1 hour and 20 minutes.

Calories **207** / Calories from fat **45** / Total fat **5.0g** / Saturated fat **0.6g** / Trans fat **0.0g** / Sodium **6mg** / Carbs **24.1g** / Sugars **14.7g** / Protein **4.5g**

Gluten-free
Low-sodium
Nightshade-free
Vegan
Vegetarian

DESSERTS

Simple Chocolate Fudge

This is an incredibly rich, creamy fudge that can be stored in the refrigerator for up to three weeks—but will probably not make it past the first week because it is addictive. The sweetness in this recipe comes from dates, so if you want to adjust the level of sweetness add or subtract the number of dates. Dates help prevent and relieve digestion problems such as constipation, and can help prevent anemia and osteoporosis.

Cooking tip This fudge can also be stored in the freezer for up to 2 months, so make a double batch. Let your fudge sit at room temperature out of the freezer for about 10 minutes to soften up before eating it.

½ cup coconut oil

¾ cup unsweetened cocoa powder

1 large ripe banana

8 dates, chopped

1 teaspoon pure vanilla extract

1. Line a 9-by-13-inch baking dish with parchment paper and set it aside.
2. In a large saucepan over medium heat, melt the coconut oil.
3. Remove the oil from the heat and stir in the cocoa powder until there are no lumps.
4. In a food processor, combine the banana, dates, and vanilla and pulse until they form a smooth paste.
5. Add the cocoa mixture to the processor and pulse until smooth and blended, scraping down the sides at least once.
6. Spoon the fudge mixture into the baking dish, cover the dish with plastic wrap, and refrigerate until the fudge is firm, about 3 hours.
7. Cut the fudge into pieces and store it in a sealed container in the refrigerator for up to 3 weeks.

Makes 24. Prep time 10 minutes. Cook time 1 minute, plus setting time.

Calories **58** / Calories from fat **44** / Total fat **4.9g** / Saturated fat **4.1g** / Trans fats **0.0g** / Sodium **1mg** / Carbs **4.9g** / Sugars **2.5g** / Protein **0.6g**

Lime Pots de Crème

This is a smooth, tart treat that can be topped with fresh berries to create a gorgeous dessert for family or guests. Buttermilk might sound heavy, but it has no butter in it. It is actually the liquid that remains after the fat is taken out of the milk to make butter. That means buttermilk has less fat than regular milk, and it's good for you because it is also a great source of calcium, phosphorus, potassium, and vitamin B_{12}.

Leftovers tip Try a tablespoon or two of buttermilk on baked potatoes (unless you are on a nightshade-free diet) to get a rich sour cream taste without all the added fat and calories.

1 cup skim milk

1 teaspoon pure vanilla extract

1 tablespoon unflavored gelatin

1 cup Greek yogurt

1 cup low-fat buttermilk

½ cup honey

Zest and juice of 1 lime

1. In a medium saucepan over medium-high heat combine the milk and vanilla.
2. Let the milk warm for about 1 minute and whisk in the gelatin.
3. Remove the milk mixture from the heat when it starts to bubble around the edges of the pan, after about 5 minutes.
4. Remove the pan from the heat and set it aside to cool for about 15 minutes.
5. In a large bowl, whisk together the remaining ingredients until very well blended.
6. Whisk the slightly cooled milk mixture into the lime mixture.
7. Spoon the mixture into four 6-ounce ramekins, cover them with plastic wrap, and put them in the refrigerator to set completely, for at least 4 hours or overnight.
8. Serve chilled.

Serves 4. Prep time 10 minutes. Cook time 7 minutes, plus setting time.

Calories **222** / Calories from fat **14** / Total fat **1.5g** / Saturated fat **1.1g** / Trans fat **0.0g** / Sodium **118mg** / Carbs **43.0g** / Sugars **42.9g** / Protein **10.7g**

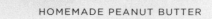

HOMEMADE PEANUT BUTTER

CHAPTER FOURTEEN

Kitchen Basics

Gluten-free
Low-fat
Low-sodium
Nightshade-free
Vegan
Vegetarian

KITCHEN
BASICS

Blueberry Chia Jam

This is not really a jam, but since you can spread it on toast and use it as a dessert topping, calling it jam does not seem like much of a culinary stretch. Blueberries are a wonderful choice for this spread, but any berry would be nice. Blueberries are very high in phytonutrients, folic acid, calcium, iron, potassium, and vitamins B_1, B_3, B_6, and C. This jam is the perfect way to start the day off with a nutritional jump.

Diet tip If your blueberries are sweet enough naturally, you can omit the maple syrup and create a lovely FODMAP-appropriate jam.

4 cups fresh blueberries
½ cup chia seeds

¼ cup pure maple syrup

1. In a food processor, combine all the ingredients and process until well blended.
2. Transfer the mixture to a medium bowl and put in the refrigerator until thickened, about 4 hours.
3. Store the jam in a sealed container in the refrigerator for up to 1 week.

Makes 16 servings. Prep time 5 minutes.

Calories **48** / Calories from fat **13** / Total fat **1.4g** / Saturated fat **0.0g** / Trans fat **0.0g** / Sodium **1mg** / Carbs **10.1g** / Sugars **6.5g** / Protein **1.0g**

Homemade Peanut Butter

Peanut butter has long been on the list for healthy eaters and people who work out or play sports, because of its high protein content. Unfortunately, processed peanut butters also contain a fair bit of sugar, salt, and preservatives. Natural peanut butter does not have to be anything other than roasted peanuts. Making it yourself will take a fair bit of time, so be patient and you will enjoy a wonderful, creamy, flavor-packed, healthy spread.

Diet tip Peanuts are certainly not a low-fat food, but the fat found in peanuts is monounsaturated fat and oleic acid, which are the same healthy fats found in olive oil.

2 cups roasted unsalted peanuts

1. In a food processor, pulse the peanuts for about 30 seconds.
2. Continue to process the peanuts in 1-minute intervals with a couple of seconds rest in between each minute to let the oils come out of the peanuts.
3. Continue to process until the peanut butter is creamy and smooth, about 20 minutes.
4. Store the peanut butter in a sealed container in the refrigerator for up to 2 weeks.

Makes 32 tablespoons. Prep time 20 minutes.

Calories **52** / Calories from fat **41** / Total fat **4.5g** / Saturated fat **0.6g** / Trans fat **0.0g** / Sodium **2mg** / Carbs **1.5g** / Sugars **0.0g** / Protein **2.4g**

Roasted Garlic

Roasted garlic is a superb addition to many clean eating recipes, as well as mashed up with potatoes or root vegetables. It has a mild, rich, almost nutty flavor. This recipe lightly blanches the garlic in milk before roasting it, to remove any bitterness that might be present. This step can be skipped with no ill effects and then the roasted garlic will be vegan.

Cooking tip You can roast the garlic in the bulb by slicing off the top to expose a little of the cloves and drizzling the whole clove with a little olive oil. Roast in the oven until the cloves are softened and then squeeze the garlic out of the papery bulb.

2 cups peeled garlic cloves
½ cup milk

1 tablespoon olive oil

1. Preheat the oven to 350°F.
2. In a small ovenproof skillet on medium-high heat, combine the garlic cloves and milk and bring to a boil.
3. Reduce the heat to low and simmer the garlic and milk for about 5 minutes, stirring occasionally.
4. Drain the milk from the skillet and stir in the olive oil.
5. Cover the skillet with foil, transfer it to the oven, and roast the garlic until it is very tender and golden, about 20 minutes.
6. Store the roasted garlic in a sealed container in the refrigerator for up to 1 week.

Serves 8. Prep time 5 minutes. Cook time 30 minutes.

Calories **25** / Calories from fat **19** / Total fat **2.1g** / Saturated fat **0.0g** / Trans fat **0.0g** / Sodium **25mg** / Carbs **1.0g** / Sugars **0.7g** / Protein **0.5g**

Spicy Lime Cilantro Dressing

Cilantro has a bright, fresh taste, and combines nicely with lime and jalapeño pepper to create a distinctive Southwestern dressing. This herb is a staple of both Latino and Asian cuisine. Cilantro is also high in many vitamins and minerals, including iron, calcium, and vitamins A, B_6, C, and K. Cilantro is used to detox the body of heavy metals, as well as to stabilize blood sugar.

Cooking tip This dressing would make a delicious marinade for fish, but remember that fish should not be marinated longer than an hour or the flesh can become tough.

¼ cup chopped fresh cilantro

2 garlic cloves

½ jalapeño pepper

¼ cup fresh lime juice

¼ cup water

Pinch of sea salt

Pinch of freshly ground black pepper

Pinch of cayenne pepper

½ cup olive oil

1. In a blender, combine all the ingredients except the oil and blend until very smooth and well combined.
2. Add the olive oil in a thin stream, and continue to blend until the dressing emulsifies.
3. Store the dressing in a sealed container in the refrigerator for up to 2 weeks.

Serves 12. Prep time 10 minutes.

Calories **73** / Calories from fat **73** / Total fat **8.4g** / Saturated fat **1.2g** / Trans fat **0.0g** / Sodium **20mg** / Carbs **0.2g** / Sugar **0.0g** / Protein **0.1g**

Yogurt Cheese

This versatile cheese should be at the top of the list of your clean eating staples. It ends up the consistency of cream cheese, and you can use it as a base for many other recipes. Add a vast assortment of other ingredients to the yogurt cheese to vary the flavor, including herbs, fruit, and chocolate.

Nutrition tip Yogurt is an excellent source of magnesium, calcium, potassium, and vitamins B_2 and B_{12}. It can help reduce the risk of high blood pressure, promote a healthy digestive system, and make you feel full.

8 cups Greek yogurt

Pinch of salt

1. Place a fine mesh sieve over a large bowl.
2. Line the sieve with 4 layers of damp cheesecloth and pour the yogurt into the sieve.
3. Cover the sieve with plastic wrap and allow the yogurt to drain overnight in the refrigerator.
4. Remove the soft cheese from the cheesecloth and store it in the refrigerator in a sealed container for up to 1 week.

Serves 8. Prep time 5 minutes, plus draining time.

Calories **169** / Calories from fat **41** / Total fat **4.5g** / Saturated fat **3.4g** / Trans fat **0.0g** / Sodium **93mg** / Carbs **9.0g** / Sugars **9.0g** / Protein **22.5g**

Cilantro Herb Salsa

Gluten-free
Low-fat
Low-sodium
Vegan
Vegetarian

KITCHEN
BASICS

Salsa is one of the most versatile staples in clean eating because you can use it for any type of meal, from breakfast to lunch wraps, and with any meat for an entrée. This is a standard mild tomato salsa with a healthy amount of pungent cilantro for flavoring. Tomatoes are available year round in most grocery stores. Try to get organic on-the-vine tomatoes for better taste and superior quality.

Cooking tip If you want a salsa that can keep for longer, try seeding your tomatoes before chopping them and reserve the scooped-out pulp for soups, sauces, and stews.

6 medium tomatoes, chopped

2 tablespoons minced garlic

1 small red onion, peeled and chopped

1 red bell pepper, seeded and finely chopped

1 small jalapeño pepper, finely chopped

½ cup chopped fresh cilantro

1. In a large bowl, mix all the ingredients together.
2. Store the salsa in a sealed container in the refrigerator for up to 3 days.

Serves 4. Prep time 10 minutes.

Calories **57** / Calories from fat **5** / Total fat **0.5g** / Saturated fat **0.0g** / Trans fat **0.0g** / Sodium **12mg** / Carbs **12.1g** / Sugars **7.0g** / Protein **2.4g**

Gluten-free
Low-sodium
Nightshade-free
Vegetarian

KITCHEN
BASICS

Lemon Garlic Vinaigrette

This vinaigrette might become your new favorite for any salad, and even an interesting dressing for a pasta dish. It has the smallest touch of honey to balance the tartness of the lemon. Honey has been a valuable culinary and medicinal ingredient for several thousand years, and continues to be used today for its warm sweetness and health benefits. It was even thought to help people live longer—and maybe it can!

Shopping tip The flavor of the honey will depend on what flowers the bees collect nectar from to make it. Try the different types to see what flavor appeals to your palate.

2 teaspoons minced garlic

¼ cup fresh lemon juice

2 tablespoons red wine vinegar

1 tablespoon chopped fresh oregano

½ teaspoon honey

Pinch of freshly ground black pepper

½ cup olive oil

1. In a small bowl, whisk together all the ingredients except the oil until well blended.
2. Whisk in the olive oil until the dressing emulsifies.
3. Store the vinaigrette in a sealed container in the refrigerator for up to 1 week.

Makes 12 tablespoons. Prep time 5 minutes.

Calories **60** / Calories from fat **57** / Total fat **6.3g** / Saturated fat **0.9g** / Trans fat **0.0g** / Sodium **16mg** / Carbs **0.7g** / Sugars **0.6g** / Protein **0.1g**

Ranch Dressing

You can use this dressing for salads and as a tasty dip for cut vegetables. The chives in this recipe add a slightly peppery taste to the dressing. Chives are one of the easiest herbs to grow and are perennials, so they continue to grow year round with a nice healthy root system. Try keeping a big pot on a sunny counter and simply snip off what you need for your recipes with a sharp pair of scissors.

Cooking tip If you want a less dense dressing, add some more buttermilk or thin it out with a touch of water.

⅔ cup low-fat buttermilk

⅓ cup plain Greek yogurt

2 tablespoons minced sweet onion

1 tablespoon chopped fresh parsley

1 tablespoon chopped fresh chives

1 teaspoon chopped fresh dill

Pinch of freshly ground black pepper

1. In a medium bowl, stir together all the ingredients until well blended.
2. Store the dressing in a sealed container in the refrigerator for up to 1 week.

Makes 16 tablespoons. Prep time 5 minutes.

Calories **8** / Calories from fat **1** / Total fat **0.1g** / Saturated fat **0.0g** / Trans fat **0.0g** / Sodium **15mg** / Carbs **0.9g** / Sugars **0.9g** / Protein **0.7g**

Tomato Pesto Vinaigrette

This is a basic vinaigrette that is perfect for everyday use on any salad. The best pesto to use in the recipe is a nice homemade one, so you know exactly what ingredients are in it. Use your own pesto recipes, or try Sun-Dried Tomato Pesto in this chapter. Use a dairy-free pesto and the vinaigrette works for vegan diets.

Cooking tip This vinaigrette is also delicious with balsamic vinegar instead of apple cider vinegar, just note that the finished product will be darker in color.

12 sun-dried tomatoes

3 tablespoons fresh lemon juice

1 tablespoon basil pesto

1 tablespoon apple cider vinegar

2 teaspoons minced garlic

Pinch of freshly ground black pepper

½ cup olive oil

1. In a blender, combine all the ingredients except the olive oil and blend into a smooth paste.
2. Add the olive oil in a thin stream while the blender is running.
3. Store the dressing in a sealed container in the refrigerator for up to 1 week.

Makes 12 tablespoons. Prep time 5 minutes.

Calories **40** / Calories from fat **38** / Total fat **4.2g** / Saturated fat **0.6g** / Trans fat **0.0g** / Sodium **21mg** / Carbs **1.4g** / Sugar **0.0g** / Protein **0.2g**

Sun-Dried Tomato Pesto

Pesto is one of the best ways to get an intense flavor into a dish without too much added fat, salt, or calories. This sun-dried tomato variation uses pecans instead of the traditional pine nuts, for a unique taste. Pecans are extremely high in antioxidants, protein, and fiber.

Leftovers tip Basil is a very delicate herb with high water content. It needs to be frozen instead of dried if you have extra. Simply put whole stems of basil in the freezer for several hours until completely frozen and then transfer them to a sealed container. Do not pack them in, because basil bruises easily.

1 cup packed fresh basil leaves

2 tablespoons chopped sun-dried tomatoes

2 tablespoons pecans

2 tablespoons grated Parmesan cheese

1 teaspoon minced garlic

Pinch of freshly ground black pepper

2 tablespoons olive oil

1. In a food processor, combine all the ingredients except the olive oil and pulse until they are well combined and form a thick paste, scraping down the sides of the bowl at least once with a spatula.
2. Add the olive oil and pulse until the oil is incorporated.
3. Store the pesto in a sealed container in the refrigerator for up to 1 week.

Makes 16 tablespoons. Prep time 10 minutes.

Calories **34** / Calories from fat **28** / Total fat **3.1g** / Saturated fat **0.8g** / Trans fat **0.0g** / Sodium **41mg** / Carbs **0.6g** / Sugar **0.0g** / Protein **1.3g**

Gluten-free
Low-fat
Low-sodium
Vegan
Vegetarian

KITCHEN
BASICS

Simple Marinara Sauce

Basil and oregano are traditional herbs in Italian cuisine, and they impart a pleasant sweetness that is mirrored in the ripe tomatoes. Basil is a great choice for this sauce; the herb has antibacterial properties.

Cooking tip Marinara sauce freezes beautifully, so whip up a double batch and store it in resealable zipper-top bags or sealed containers for up to a year in the freezer.

½ small sweet onion, peeled and chopped
1 tablespoon minced garlic
1 teaspoon olive oil
6 large tomatoes, coarsely chopped
½ cup water

1 small bay leaf
3 tablespoons chopped fresh basil
1 tablespoon chopped fresh oregano
Pinch of freshly ground black pepper

1. In a large saucepan over medium heat, sauté the onion and garlic in the oil until softened and lightly browned, about 10 minutes.
2. Add the tomatoes, water, and bay leaf and bring the mixture to a gentle boil.
3. Reduce the heat to low and simmer, covered, for about 15 minutes.
4. Remove the pan from the heat and take out the bay leaf.
5. Stir in the basil, oregano, and pepper.
6. Serve immediately or chill and store the sauce in the refrigerator in a sealed container for up to 1 week.

Serves 4. Prep time 5 minutes. Cook time 25 minutes.

Calories **70** / Calories from fat **17** / Total fat **1.9g** / Saturated fat **0.0g** / Trans fat **0.0g** / Sodium **14mg** / Carbs **13.0g** / Sugars **7.6g** / Protein **2.8g**

Tzatziki Sauce

Gluten-free
Low-fat
Nightshade-free
Vegetarian

KITCHEN
BASICS

If you have ever tried gyros or souvlaki, you've tasted this tangy, rich sauce. It's a great complement to both meats and vegetables. The garlic, a common ingredient in almost every cuisine in the world, adds a wonderful pungent flavor. To get the freshest garlic, try to buy bulbs that feel heavy, because this means they are not old and dried out.

Cooking tip Sometimes it is impossible to get the scent of garlic off your hands after you mince it. Try rubbing something stainless steel over your hands, like a spoon or the side of a bowl, to remove the smell. Or simply run your hands along your stainless steel sink.

2 cups plain Greek yogurt
1 large English cucumber, grated, with all
  the liquid squeezed out

3 tablespoons chopped fresh dill
1 teaspoon minced garlic
Pinch of sea salt

1. In a medium bowl, stir together all the ingredients until they are well blended.
2. Store the sauce in a sealed container in the refrigerator for up to 4 days.

Makes 32 tablespoons. Prep time 5 minutes.

Calories **14** / Calories from fat **5** / Total fat **0.6g** / Saturated fat **0.0g** / Trans fat **0.0g** / Sodium **13mg** / Carbs **1.1g** / Sugar **0.6g** / Protein **1.4g**

FODMAP-free
Gluten-free
Nightshade-free
Vegetarian

KITCHEN
BASICS

Clean Eating Mayonnaise

This is not a truly healthy recipe, but it is much better than processed mayonnaise, which has additives and preservatives. Eating clean is all about food choices that are not processed, and this tangy dressing fits those guidelines. Eat this spread and dressing sparingly with sandwiches or wraps, and use it as a base for your favorite dips as a rare treat.

Shopping tip While traditional mayonnaise is made with raw egg yolks, that's not really a safe option due to the risk of salmonella infection. Eggs can be pasteurized in the shell or sold in cartons of liquid pasteurized egg. Pasteurization involves nothing but heat, so it does not alter the egg's nutrition.

2 yolks from pasteurized eggs or ⅓ cup
    pasteurized liquid eggs
2 teaspoons white wine vinegar
2 teaspoons Dijon mustard

½ teaspoon sea salt
¼ teaspoon freshly ground black pepper
1 cup olive oil

1. In a blender, combine the eggs, vinegar, mustard, salt, and pepper until well mixed.
2. Run the blender on low speed and slowly add approximately one-third of the oil in a thin stream, until the mixture is creamy.
3. Add the remaining oil in a thin stream until it is completely incorporated and the mayonnaise is thick.
4. Transfer the mayonnaise to a sealed container and store it in the refrigerator for up to 2 weeks.

Makes 32 teaspoons. Prep time 5 minutes.

Calories **58** / Calories from fat **58** / Total fat **6.6g** / Saturated fat **1.0g** / Trans fat **0.0g** / Sodium **35mg** / Carbs **0.1g** / Sugar **0.0g** / Protein **0.2g**

Cinnamon Applesauce

Most of the applesauce found on grocery store shelves doesn't really taste like apples and has an incredible array of added ingredients. Since making your own is so simple, there is no need to ever use store-bought again for your breakfast, snacks, desserts, and baked goods. Make a big batch, because this applesauce keeps well in the freezer.

Cooking tip If you have a slow cooker, one of the best ways to cook applesauce is to place all your ingredients into the slow cooker, and cook them on low until you have the desired texture.

6 apples, peeled, cored, and chopped into
   ½-inch chunks
½ cup water

1 teaspoon fresh lemon juice
1 teaspoon ground cinnamon

1. In a medium saucepan over medium-high heat, combine the apples, water, and lemon juice and bring to a boil.
2. Reduce the heat to low and simmer until the apples are tender, about 15 minutes.
3. Remove the mixture from the heat and either mash the apples with a potato masher or use an immersion blender to purée, depending on how chunky you want the finished product.
4. Stir in the cinnamon and serve either warm or cold.
5. Store the applesauce in the refrigerator in a sealed container for up to 1 week.

Serves 4. Prep time 5 minutes. Cook time 15 minutes.

Calories **144** / Calories from fat **0** / Total fat **0.0g** / Saturated fat **0.0g** / Trans fat **0.0g** / Sodium **4mg** / Carbs **32.8g** / Sugars **28.4g** / Protein **0.0g**

Appendix

Grab 'n Go: Thirty-Five Clean Eating Snack Ideas

1. Nuts, dried fruit, seeds, and trail mix

2. Fresh fruit (plain, or with Greek yogurt)

3. Fresh vegetables

4. Hardboiled eggs

5. Greek yogurt with granola or nuts

6. Smoothies

7. Frozen grapes

8. Homemade unsweetened applesauce

9. Apple slices with natural nut butters

10. Air-popped popcorn

11. Edamame

12. Celery sticks topped with natural peanut butter and raisins

13. Homemade fruit popsicles

14. Medjool dates

15. Dried fruit or vegetable chips

16. Mixed green salad

17. Steel-cut oatmeal with a little homemade applesauce

18. Homemade baked sweet potato fries

19. Homemade protein bar

20. Baked pita bread with honey and dried fruit

21. Rye melba toast with low-fat cream cheese and dried cranberries

22. One ounce of great quality dark chocolate

23. Half a whole-wheat English muffin with nut butter

24. Wraps stuffed with leftovers

25. Apples with cheese

26. Whole-wheat pretzels

27. Homemade fruit leathers

28. 100 percent shredded wheat with low-fat almond milk

29. Homemade clean eating cookies or muffins

30. One can of water-packed tuna with a drizzle of homemade dressing

31. Half an avocado with homemade salsa

32. Chickpeas, either plain or roasted

33. Wraps and pitas stuffed with lean meats, veggies, and beans

34. Homemade beef jerky

35. Olives and low-sodium pickles

The Dirty Dozen Plus

As you probably already know, not all produce is created equal, but some fruits and vegetables are cleaner than others. The dirty dozen are fruits and vegetables the Environmental Working Group (EWG) has identified as being the most contaminated. To steer clear of hazardous pesticides, choose organic when buying the produce on this list. Visit the Environmental Working Group's website at www.ewg.org for updates to this list.

- Apples
- Celery
- Cherry tomatoes
- Cucumbers
- Grapes
- Hot peppers

- Kale/collard greens
- Nectarines (imported)
- Peaches
- Potatoes
- Snap peas (imported)
- Spinach
- Sweet bell peppers
- Strawberries

The Clean Fifteen

The clean fifteen are nonorganic fruits and vegetables the EWG has identified as having the least amount of contamination. If you're watching your food budget, the clean fifteen are the best produce to buy nonorganic. Visit the Environmental Working Group's website at www.ewg.org for updates to this list.

- Asparagus
- Avocados
- Cabbage
- Cantaloupe
- Eggplant
- Grapefruit
- Kiwis
- Mangoes
- Mushrooms
- Onions
- Papayas
- Pineapple
- Sweet corn
- Sweet peas (frozen)
- Sweet potatoes

Glossary

amino acids there are twenty amino acids, which are the building blocks of protein. The body uses the protein from food by breaking it down into amino acids.

antioxidants the vitamins, minerals, and phytonutrients that protect your body from free radicals and are crucial for good health.

artificial sweeteners laboratory-created sweeteners created to replace sugar. These are not on the clean eating plan.

blood glucose or blood sugar the glucose (sugar) level in the blood.

calories a unit of energy. With respect to food, calories are the amount of energy in the food; the higher the number, the more energy the food contains.

carbohydrates organic compounds comprised of sugars, starches, and cellulose. The body breaks down carbohydrates into blood sugar, which is used as energy. Carbohydrates can be simple or complex. Simple carbohydrates are not recommended on a clean eating diet because they are broken down very quickly, creating spikes in blood sugar. Complex carbohydrates include many of the foods found in the clean eating diet, such as vegetables, fruit, whole grains, and legumes. These healthy carbs break down more slowly, for more stable blood sugar.

chia seeds nutritious seeds with the highest level of omega-3 fatty acids found in a plant source. They are a member of the mint family, and are often used in sauces or puddings because they can soak up about nine times their volume in liquid.

coconut oil an oil that comes from coconut milk. It is high in saturated fat but also has many health benefits, so it is part of the clean eating plan. Coconut oil supports a healthy digestive system, boosts immunity, and helps lower cholesterol.

complete proteins proteins that contain all nine essential amino acids. Essential amino acids cannot be produced in the body so they need to come from foods such as dairy, meats, poultry, and seafood.

diet the food you eat—although the word is often applied to weight loss or health oriented eating plans.

essential amino acids the nine amino acids that the body cannot produce in the quantities required, or at all.

essential fatty acids the most well-known essential fatty acids are omega-3s and omega-6s. These fats are not produced in the body and need to be taken from food, because they are crucial for proper physical functioning.

fiber the indigestible component in plants that sweeps through the body like a broom. It is crucial for a healthy, efficient digestive system. A diet high in fiber can help prevent some types of cancer, diabetes, heart disease, and other health problems.

flavonoids natural pigments found in plants that function as antioxidants to help protect human cells from damage.

flaxseed the seeds of the flax plant; they are a great plant source of omega-3 fatty acids, and are very high in fiber and other nutrients.

free radicals oxygen or nitrogen molecules that are missing electrons, so they try to take electrons from the cells in the body, causing damage. Unchecked, free radicals can damage cells in all kinds of ways.

gluten a cereal grain protein that can cause health problems in people with gluten sensitivity.

glycemic index a measure of how fast a food causes the blood sugar to rise after consuming it.

grass-fed meat the recommended meat on the clean eating plan because it is not factory-farmed and comes from pasture-raised animals that are allowed to graze.

insulin the hormone that moves glucose from the blood into the cells.

lactose a sugar in milk that can be an allergen for many people.

macronutrients main groups of nutrients that your body uses for essential tasks; they include protein, carbohydrates, and fat.

omega-3 fatty acid a family of three fats (ALA, EPA, and DHA) that are not produced in the body but are essential for health because omega-3s help with almost every type of cell activity.

omega-6 fatty acid unsaturated fatty acids that aren't made by the body but are crucial for good health.

phytonutrients beneficial compounds found only in plants and may help prevent disease and keep your body functioning smoothly.

prebiotics indigestible carbohydrates that serve as food for probiotics.

probiotics the bacteria that live in your digestive system that help digestion and aid in eliminating bad bacteria from the body.

processed foods products treated with additives, chemicals, and preservatives; these foods are not recommended when eating clean.

protein essential nutrient made from amino acids that is used for many body functions, and maintaining and building cells.

References

Collins, Sonya. "The Truth About Belly Fat." WebMD. Accessed March 9, 2014. http://www.webmd.com/diet/features/the-truth-about-belly-fat.

dLife. "12 Best Fiber Foods." Accessed March 9, 2014. http://www.dlife.com/dlife_media/diabetes_slideshows/12-best-fiber-foods?index=9.

Environmental Working Group. "EWG's 2013 Shopper's Guide to Pesticides in Produce." Accessed March 9, 2014. http://www.ewg.org/foodnews/summary.php.

Environmental Working Group. "PCBs in Farmed Salmon." Accessed March 9, 2014. http://www.ewg.org/reports/farmedpcbs.

Goto, K., et al. "Effects of resistance exercise on lipolysis during subsequent submaximal exercise." *Medicine & Science in Sports & Exercise.* February 2007; 39(2): 308–15.

Harvard School of Public Health. "Fiber: Start Roughing It!" The Nutrition Source. Accessed March 9, 2014. http://www.hsph.harvard.edu/nutritionsource/what-should-you-eat/fiber-full-story/.

Hensrud, Donald, MD. "Sleep and Weight Gain: What's the Connection?" Mayo Clinic. Accessed March 9, 2014. http://www.mayoclinic.com/health/sleep-and-weight-gain/AN02178/.

Hyman, Mark, MD. *The Blood Sugar Solution.* New York: Little, Brown and Company, 2012.

Jacob, Agalee. "Damaging Effects of Too Much Sugar in the Diet." SF Gate, Healthy Eating. Accessed March 9, 2014. http://healthyeating.sfgate.com/damaging-effects-much-sugar-diet-1508.html.

Mayo Clinic Staff. "Exercise: 7 benefits of regular physical activity." Accessed March 9, 2014. http://www.mayoclinic.com/health/exercise/HQ01676.

Mckee, G. *Guide to Food Additives.* Chicago: The Learning Seed, 2008.

MediResource Canada. "High Cholesterol." Accessed March 9, 2014. http://bodyandhealth
.canada.com/channel_condition_info_details.asp?disease_id=148&channel_id
=41&relation_id=10852.

National Cancer Institute. "Cruciferous Vegetables and Cancer Prevention." Accessed March
9, 2014. http://www.cancer.gov/cancertopics/factsheet/diet/cruciferous-vegetables.

Natural Resources Defense Council. "Consumer Guide to Mercury in Fish." Accessed March
9, 2014. http://www.nrdc.org/health/effects/mercury/guide.asp.

Reno, Tosca. *The Eat-Clean Diet: Fast Fat-Loss That Lasts Forever!* Mississauga, Ontario:
Robert Kennedy Publishing, 2007.

Teicholz, Nina. "What If Bad Fat Is Actually Good for You?" *Men's Health.* October 10, 2007.
Accessed March 9, 2014. http://www.menshealth.com/health/saturated-fat?fullpage=true.

Tomiyama, Janet A., et al. "Low Calorie Dieting Increases Cortisol," *Psychosomatic Medicine.*
May 2010; 72(4): 357–364.

Venuto, Tom. *The Body Fat Solution.* New York: Avery, 2009.

WebMD. "Portion Control and Weight Loss." Accessed March 9, 2014. http://www.webmd.com
/diet/control-portion-size.

Wedro, Benjamin, MD. "High Cholesterol." eMedicine Health. Accessed March 9, 2014.
http://www.emedicinehealth.com/high_cholesterol/article_em.htm.

Women Fitness. "Ugly Truths About White Flour." Accessed March 9, 2014.
http://www.womenfitness.net/ugly_truths.htm.

Worden, Jeni, GP. "Carbohydrates." NetDoctor. Accessed March 9, 2014. http://www.netdoctor
.co.uk/focus/nutrition/facts/lifestylemanagement/carbohydrates.htm.

Recipe Index

Subject Index

CPSIA information can be obtained at www.ICGtesting.com
Printed in the USA
LVOW01*1529110914

403629LV00003B/5/P